"We are physically and mentally what we eat and what we think."

Edgar Cayce's approach to diet and health was based on his concepts of the body as the temple of the soul— and the union between our physical selves, our eternal souls and the eternal energy that surrounds us. In this practical, everyday guide to better living, three Edgar Cayce students have compiled complete menus, recipes, and dietary guidelines based on the Cayce Readings. Here are answers to hundreds of questions, including:

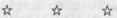

- Is there such a thing as "proper" food combining?
- What is the importance of acidity and alkalinity in the diet?
- Is it healthy to eat meat?
- What is the most nutritious way to cook vegetables?
- Can food affect your moods and psychological well-being?

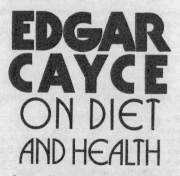

EDGAR CAYCE ON DIET AND HEALTH

is a vital companion to your new, healthier life.

Books in
The Edgar Cayce Series

THERE WILL YOUR HEART BE ALSO
DREAMS YOUR MAGIC MIRROR
EDGAR CAYCE ON DIET AND HEALTH
EDGAR CAYCE ON HEALING
DREAMS IN THE LIFE OF PRAYER
EDGAR CAYCE ON RELIGION AND
PSYCHIC EXPERIENCE
EDGAR CAYCE ON ESP
THE EDGAR CAYCE READER
EDGAR CAYCE ON ATLANTIS
THE EDGAR CAYCE READER #2
EDGAR CAYCE ON DREAMS
EDGAR CAYCE ON PROPHECY
EDGAR CAYCE ON REINCARNATION
EDGAR CAYCE ON JESUS AND HIS CHURCH
EDGAR CAYCE ON THE DEAD SEA SCROLLS
EDGAR CAYCE ENCYCLOPEDIA OF HEALING
EDGAR CAYCE ON MYSTERIES OF THE MIND*
YOU CAN REMEMBER YOUR PAST LIVES*
EDGAR CAYCE ON THE POWER OF COLOR, STONES AND CRYSTALS*
EDGAR CAYCE ANSWERS LIFE'S 10
MOST IMPORTANT QUESTIONS*
EDGAR CAYCE ON SECRETS OF THE UNIVERSE AND HOW
TO USE THEM IN YOUR LIFE*

Published by
WARNER BOOKS   *forthcoming

EDGAR CAYCE
ON DIET
AND HEALTH

BY ANNE READ,
CAROL ILSTRUP AND
MARGARET GAMMON
UNDER THE EDITORSHIP OF
HUGH LYNN CAYCE
Director, Association for Research and Enlightenment

WARNER BOOKS

A Warner Communications Company

WARNER BOOKS EDITION

Warner Books, Inc.
666 Fifth Avenue
New York, N.Y. 10103

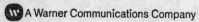 A Warner Communications Company

Printed in the United States of America

First Printing: March, 1969

Reissued: October, 1988

20   19   18

CONTENTS

INTRODUCTION

WHO WAS EDGAR CAYCE?

The eleven books which have been written about him have totaled more than a million in sales, and more than ten other books have devoted sections to his life and talents. He has been featured in dozens of magazines and hundreds of newspaper articles dating from 1900 to the present. What was so unique about him?

It depends upon through whose eyes you look at him. A goodly number of his contemporaries knew the "waking" Edgar Cayce as a gifted professional photographer. Another cross section (predominantly children) admired him as a warm and friendly Sunday School teacher. His own family knew him as a wonderful husband and father.

The "sleeping" Edgar Cayce was an entirely different figure; a psychic known to thousands of people, in all walks of life, who had cause to be grateful for his help; indeed, many of them believe that he alone had either saved or changed their lives when all seemed lost. The "sleeping" Edgar Cayce was a medical diagnostician, a prophet, and a devoted proponent of Bible lore.

In June 1954, the University of Chicago held him in sufficient respect to accept a Ph.D. thesis based on a study of his life and work: in this thesis the graduate referred to him as a "religious seer." In June of that same year, the children's comic book *House of Mystery* bestowed on him the impressive title of "America's Most Mysterious Man!"

Even as a child on a farm near Hopkinsville, Kentucky, where he was born on March 18, 1877, Edgar Cayce displayed powers of perception which seemed to extend beyond the normal range of the five senses. At the age of six or seven he told his parents that he was able to see and talk to "visions," sometimes of relatives who had recently died. His parents attributed this to the overactive imagination of a lonely child who had been influenced by the dramatic language of the revival meetings which were popular in that section of the country. Later, by sleeping with his head on his schoolbooks, he developed some form of photographic memory, which helped him advance rapidly in the country school. This faded, however, and Edgar completed only his seventh grade before he sought his own place in the world.

By twenty-one he had become the salesman for a wholesale stationery company. At this time he developed a gradual paralysis of the throat muscles, which threatened the loss of his voice. When doctors were unable to find a physical cause for these conditions, hypnosis was tried, but failed to have any permanent effect.

As a last resort, Edgar asked a friend to help him re-enter the same kind of hypnotic sleep that had enabled him to memorize his schoolbooks as a child. His friend gave him the necessary suggestion, and once he was in self-induced trance, Edgar came to grips with his own problem. He recommended medication and manipulative therapy which successfully restored his voice and repaired his system.

A group of physicians from Hopkinsville and Bowling Green, Kentucky, took advantage of his unique talent to diagnose their own patients. They soon discovered that Cayce only needed to be given the name and address of the patient, wherever he was, and was then able to "tune in" telepathically on that individual's mind and body as easily as if they were both in the same room. He needed, and was given, no other information regarding any patient.

One of the young M.D.'s, Dr. Wesley Ketchum, submitted a report on this unorthodox procedure to a clinical research society in Boston. On October 9, 1910, *The New York Times* carried two pages of headlines and pictures. From that day on, invalids from all over the country sought help from the "Wonder Man."

When Edgar Cayce died on January 3, 1945, in Virginia Beach, Virginia, he left well over fourteen thousand documented stenographic records of the telepathic-clairvoyant statements he had given for more than eight thousand different people over a period of forty-three years. These typewritten documents are referred to as "readings."

These readings constitute one of the largest and most im-

8

pressive records of psychic perception ever to emanate from a single individual. Together with their relevant records, correspondence and reports, they had been cross-indexed under thousands of subject-headings and placed at the disposal of psychologists, students, writers and investigators who come in increasing numbers to examine them.

A foundation known as the A.R.E. (The Association for Research and Enlightenment, Inc., P.O. Box 595, Virginia Beach, Virginia, 23451) was created in 1932 to preserve these readings. As an open-membership research society, it continues to index and catalogue the information, initiate investigation and experiments, and promote conference, seminars and lectures. Until now its published findings have been made available to its members through its own publishing facilities.

Now Paperback Library has made it possible to present a series of popular volumes dealing with those subjects from the Edgar Cayce readings most likely to appeal to public interest.

In this volume we have some of the most practical data to be found in the Edgar Cayce readings. Three people, Margaret Gammon, Carol Ilstrup and Anne Read, have cooperated to put together *Edgar Cayce on Diet and Health*. Diet, from Edgar's Cayce's point of view, is one of the essential considerations for happiness in an experience on Earth. His central theme is "The body is the temple of the soul." In a healthy body the soul is capable of greater service in most instances. His ideas for the development of greater sensitivity (increased ESP capacities) should be considered also. After you have adjusted to these suggestions for a more balanced diet for six months to a year you may be interested in more detailed studies of the special diets for greater psychic awareness—at that point get in touch with the Association.

—HUGH LYNN CAYCE

FOREWORD

The arrangement of this material and commentaries on it have been made by one who has been in food work for over fifteen years, and closely associated with nutritionists as well as the body of literature which daily comes to their desks to keep their knowledge up to date. A wealth of material has been available for correlation with the Edgar Cayce dietary data, but only a small proportion could be included here.

Almost all who consulted Edgar Cayce for physical readings (indicated in the text by "P" followed by the number recorded in the files at Virginia Beach) were given dietary suggestions, voluntarily or by request. Many who requested Life Readings (indicated by "L" and a file number) were also given directions for proper food suitable to the individual. This fact confirms the extraordinary scope of wisdom by which the body-mind-soul is seen to be interrelated, and the food intake an important factor in the whole. All dietary suggestions from readings for people with disease or physical ailments—even that of constipation or overweight, common as they are—have, however, been eliminated in this booklet. Instead, selections have been made from the large body of information about the normal diet, or diet for normal people. Other information is available to members of the Association for Research and Enlightenment, at Virginia Beach.

In compiling this material from the Edgar Cayce readings, one is immediately struck by the high degree of conformance with the best of modern dietetic opinion—if one includes *research* and *trends of research*.

There is, of course, some disagreement. There is also disagreement between various findings of modern research.

One set may contradict another, yet in the overall view even the most dedicated scientist holds a faith that the truth will eventually emerge, that apparently contradictory information will eventually be harmonized if it contains truth. The scientific attitude is that of "wait and see."

Just so, we also are inclined to wait and see. Meantime, we accept the information from the Edgar Cayce readings because in thousands of instances it proved beneficial and practical.

CHAPTER 1: PHILOSOPHY

Psychosomatic medicine is the new "discovery" by the medical profession, by which a connection between mental attitude and bodily health is now acknowledged and even made respectable.

In the readings by Edgar Cayce, this spiritual and mental life are not separated from the physical. All three are one, the readings gave. The importance of treating the body considerately, even reverently, since it is the temple of the spirit, is stressed over and over again in the readings.

> The body of each entity is the temple of the living God. To live—to be—and to maintain bodily activity unto the glory of the Creative Forces—is the purpose of the entrance of each entity into material consciousness.
>
> 2981-L-1

> Study those charts pertaining to keeping well-balanced in the chemical forces of the body. Not in such a way as to become a human pillbox, but rather to know the law and to keep it.   2981-P-2

> There is as much of God in the physical as there is in the spiritual or mental, for it should be one!   69-P

> Each soul is the temple of the living God. Thus be more mindful of the body for the body's sake, that it may be a better channel for manifesting spiritual truths.
>
> 2938-L-1

> Urges arise, then, not only from what one eats, but from what one thinks—and from what one does about what one thinks and eats! Also from what one digests mentally and spiritually.   2533-L-4

13

Mind is ever the builder. That which the body-mind feeds upon is what it gradually becomes, *providing assimilation takes place.* Just as in the physical body digestion does not necessarily mean assimilation; neither in the mental body does it means that what is read, heard or spoken to the body is assimilated by the mental body.   3102-P-1

Interrelationships of nutritional factors in the body, as they pertain to assimilation and digestion, constitute an area in which scientists themselves admit lack of information and need for more light.

W.H. Sebrell, Jr., M.D., Director of the National Institute of Health, U.S. Public Health Service, discussed the relationship of these factors in a welcoming address before the National Food and Nutrition Institute in Washington, D.C. Dr. Sebrell lists these questions which call for answers:

1. How do the more than 50 presently known essential nutrients work in the healthy and sick organism?

2. How well does the individual utilize his food?

3. What is the interrelationship of nutrients in the body?

Dr. Sebrell poses two more questions that relate to the preceding three:

4. When and to what extent is *appetite* reliable in the selection of a balanced diet?

5. How often should the body get specific nutrients and in what relation to one another? The time factor may be more important than is now realized.

The fourth question will remind the reader of the "Appestat," a control area for appetite, located in the brain; a term first used by Dr. Norman Jolliffe in his book, *Reduce and Stay Reduced.* In the psychosomatic approach to the problem of obesity, the reason given for overeating is to obtain

14

emotional satisfaction. The Cayce Readings also have something to say on this point.

The body should keep that diet which the physical *needs* through its inmost desires, and not override those conditions by the will of the individual. For the inmost desires of the individual would—and do lead this physical body correctly. . . . It is only when these are *overridden* by self-aggrandizement, or when self's motives are for carnal excess or success of the physical—that the body becomes *enamored* with things that hinder it. Hold steady along the lines which lead to understanding of self, and so present the physical body that it may be holy and acceptable unto Him. Remember that the physical is the earthly temple of God, to whom one should give the very best. It is only a reasonable service that this be done.   257-P-3

What effect have the emotions upon digestion and assimiliation? A direct effect, the readings declared:

Be mindful of the diet that it is kept proper. Take time to eat and to eat the right thing. Then give time for the digestive forces to act, before becoming so mentally and bodily active as to upset the digestion.   243-P-17

True, the body should eat, and should eat slowly; yet when worried, overtaxed, or when the body cannot make a business of eating but is eating merely to pass away the time, or just to fill up time—it is not good. For, the food will not digest, as the body sees.   900-D-311,2

Especially with this body, there should not be any food taken when the body is over-wrought in any way—whether caused from high-strung conditions, from wrath, or from depression of any kind. It is preferable at such times to take water or buttermilk. Never take sweet milk under such conditions.   243-P-4,5

It is a great detriment to better physical functioning to overload the stomach when the body is worried or under any general strain. Equally bad for the body is to take

15

foods whether or not there is felt the need or desire for
them. 277-P-1

Never when under strain, very tired, very excited, or
very mad should the body take foods into the system.
And never take any food that the body finds is not agree-
ing with same. 137-D-15

CHAPTER 2: "FROM THE READINGS"

"The body is the temple of the living God." This idea, told repeatedly in the Bible, is reiterated and enlarged upon throughout the Cayce readings. If we would keep that temple in such a condition as to glorify the Maker, it is imperative that we learn and adhere to certain laws, certain rules in regard to the nutritional needs of the body. For,

> We are, physically and mentally, what we eat and what we think.   288-38

Vitamins and Minerals

The need for vitamins and minerals is now widely recognized, as is much concerning their functions and sources. The readings, however, add a great deal to our understanding of these and how they may be supplied. Vitamins, one reading explains, are

> the Creative Forces working with body energies for the renewing of the body.   3511-1

Another explains that they are food for the glands, or

> that from which the glands take those necessary influences to supply the energies to enable the various organs of the body to reproduce themselves.   2072-9

The glands, it is further explained, control the supply of materials for rebuilding or reproducing the various tissues in the body, while vitamins are elements or forces required for enabling each organ to carry on in its creative function or generative activity.

17

The readings supply some little-recognized facts concerning functions of various vitamins: for example, Vitamin A in addition to other functions, is important for nerves, bone and the brain force; B, in addition to facilitating the functioning of the nerves, also supplies

> to the chyle that ability for it to control the influence of fats, which is necessary . . . to carry on the reproducing of the oils that prevent the tenseness in the joints, or that prevent the joints from becoming atrophied or dry, or to creak. 2072-9

They also say that a part of the function of C is to supply

> the necessary influences to the flexes of every nature throughout the body, whether of a muscular or tendon nature, or a heart reaction, or a kidney contraction, the batting of the eye or the supplying of the saliva and the muscular forces in face. 2072-9

and that a C deficiency results in

> bad eliminations from the incoordination of the excretory functioning of the alimentary canal, as well as the heart, liver and lungs, through the expelling of those forces that are a part of the structural portion of the body. 2072-9

From the foregoing it would seem that the vitamins may be even more important than we had realized, but we are told also that vitamins are only a combination of basic elements already found in the body,

> give a name, mostly for confusion, by those who would tell you what to do for a price. 2533-6

and we are then warned against taking supplementary vitamins over long periods of time, lest the body, if it comes to rely upon these, cease to produce them in the body, even though the food values are kept balanced. Conversely, there may be an over-abundance of vitamins, and unless

18

activities physical of the body are such as to put same into activity they become as drosses and set themselves to become operative irrespective of other conditions.

341-31

In such cases these unused vitamins act very much as bacilli and are destructive to tissue, affecting the plasma of the blood supply or the emunctory and lymph.

In most instances the readings agree with accepted dietary opinion as to which foods are rich in vitamins—and among the fruits and vegetables especially, those that are yellow in color—yellow peaches and apples, squashes, carrots, citrus fruits, etc. They add, however, some facts not generally recognized:

Quite a dissertation might be given as to the effect of tomatoes upon the human system. Of all the vegetables, tomatoes carry most of the vitamins in a well-balanced assimilative manner for the activities in the system. Yet if these are not cared for properly, they may become very destructive to a physical organism, that is, if they ripen after being pulled, or if there is the contamination with other influences . . . The tomato is one vegetable that in most instances (because of the greater uniform activity) is preferable to be eaten after being canned, for it is then much more uniform.

584-5

The value of gelatin in the diet is recognized, but the reasons for its benefits have been somewhat of a puzzle to nutritionists, since the amount of energy it supplies is out of proportion to the caloric value of its known elements. The readings give this explanation:

It isn't the vitamin content [in gelatin] but it is ability to work with the activities of the glands, causing the glands to take from that absorbed or digested the vitamins that would not be active if there is not sufficient gelatin in the body . . . There may be mixed with any chemical, that which makes the rest of the system susceptible or able to call from the system that needed. It becomes, then, as

19

it were, 'sensitive' to conditions. Without it [the gelatin] there is not that sensitivity.   849-75

Methods of preparing food may preserve or destroy much of the vitamin content. Thus fresh foods should, of course, be used as fresh as possible. Frozen vegetables, the readings say, have usually lost much of their vitamin content

> unless there is the reinforcement in them when they are either prepared for food or when frozen.

There is the possibility, of course, that this was true only of the slow-freezing methods of that time (year 1942) and may not hold true with the flash-freezing methods used commercially at present. Fruits, however, it is stated, lose little of their vitamin content by freezing. Cooking foods quickly by the steam pressure method, the readings relate, preserves the vitamins. (Contrary to some nutritional opinions.) (See 462-14 and 340-31.) Also recommended is cooking in Patapar paper, a parchment paper, in order to preserve the juices containing much of the vitamin value. (See 1963-2 and 1196-7.) One reading, emphasizing the need for more Vitamin B-1, said:

> All of the vegetables cooked in their own juices, and the body eating the juices with same.   2529-1

The need for certain minerals was given in numerous readings. Often mentioned are calcium, phosphorus, and iron. While all the minerals are undoubtedly of importance, these were evidently most often found to be insufficient in the diets of those for whom physical readings were given, and we may assume that they are often lacking in the average diet.

> Keep plenty of those foods that supply calcium to the body. These we would find especially in raw carrots, cooked turnips and turnip greens, all characters of salads—especially as of water cress, mustard and the like—these especially taken raw.   1968-6

When there is fowl taken—that is of chicken, goose, duck, turkey or the like—chew the bony pieces or make broths of them. 808-15 Milk and milk products rich in calcium are highly recommended.

One individual was told:

Preferably the raw milk, if it is certified milk. 275-25

Another reading, given 1/17/44, for a two-year-old child, warned, however:

Raw milk—provided it is from cows that don't eat certain characters of food. If they eat dry food, it is well. If they eat certain types of weeds or grass grown this time of year, it won't be so good for the body. 2752-3

The phosphorus forming foods are principally carrots, lettuce, (rather the leaf lettuce, which has more soporific activity than the head lettuce), shell fish, salsify, the peelings of Irish potatoes, and things of such natures . . . Citrus fruit juices, plenty of milk, the Bulgarian buttermilk (Yogurt) is the better . . . or the fresh milk that is warm with animal heat, which carries more of the phosphorus. 560-2

Let the iron be rather taken in the foods (instead of from medicinal sources) as it is more easily assimilated from the vegetable forces. 1187-9

Foods high in iron are spinach, lentils, red cabbage, berries, raisins, liver, grapes, pears, onions and asparagus.

Concerning sources of minerals in general, or in combination, these are given:

Cereals that carry the heart of the grain, vegetables of the leafy kind, fruit and nuts. 1131-2

Rolled or cracked wheat, not cooked too long, is recommended to

add to the body the proper proportions of iron, silicon and vitamins necessary to build up the blood supply that makes for resistance in the system. 840-1

And the almond (recommended in several readings to guard against or counteract a tendency toward cancer)

carries more phosphorus and iron in a combination
easily assimilated than any other nut.   1131-2

PHYSIOLOGICAL EFFECTS OF FOODS

In recommending specific foods, the readings attributed to them certain physiological effects. Some of these may be due to little-understood effects of the vitamins they contain; others apparently have effects aside from vitamin or mineral content.

Raw green peppers are better in combinations than by
themselves. Their tendency is for an activity to the
pylorus; not the activity in the pylorus itself, but more in
the activity from the flow of the pylorus to the churning
effect upon the duodenum in its digestion. Hence it is an
activity for digestive forces. Peppers, then, taken with
green cabbage, lettuce, are very good for this body, taken
in moderation.   404-6

Beef juice taken in small sips, more than one person was told,

will work toward producing the gastric flow through
the intestinal system; first, in the salivary reactions to the
very nature of the properties themselves; second, with the
gastric flow from the upper portions of the stomach or
through the cardiac reaction at the end of the esophagus
that produces the first of the lacteal's reaction to the
gastric flows in the stomach or digestive forces themselves; thirdly, making for an activity through the
pylorus and the duodenum that becomes stimulating to
the activity of the flows without producing the tendencies for accumulation of gases.   1100-10

Meats, especially glandular meats such as calf's liver, brains and tripe, were advised for their "blood-building properties." More often, however, "Fish, fowl, and lamb, never fried," were recommended. Fowl prepared in such a way that "more of the bone structure itself" is used was given, not only for the actual calcium content of the bones but also "that better reaction for the assimilation of calcium through the system is obtained." 1523-8

Another reading (5069-1) also stated that "chewing the bones will be worth more to the body in strengthening and in the eliminations" and added that when these are stewed the lid should be kept on so that "the boiling will not carry off that which is best to be taken."

Cooked long enough in a pressure cooker, the bones become dissolved.

Certain vegetables were recommended for their effect in protecting the body against communicable diseases.

Plenty of lettuce should always be eaten by almost everybody; for this supplies an effluvium in the blood stream itself that is a destructive force to most of those influences that attack the blood stream. It's a purifier.
404-6

Raw vegetables, such as tomatoes, lettuce, celery, spinach, carrots, beet tops, mustard greens and onions were said to

make for the purifying of the humour in the lymph blood—as this is absorbed by the lacteal ducts as it is digested. 340-1

Cooked onions and beets were also said to be blood purifiers.

A food which can be used to "cleanse all toxic forces from any system" is "raw apples when taken alone, no other food for three days, then followed with olive oil. (Half a cup)"
820-2

Raw apples, under other circumstances, however, were advised against, unless eaten, say, between meals with no other food. (See 820-2 & 567-7.)

That portion of carrots close to the top carries "the vital

23

energies which stimulate the optic reactions between kidneys and the optics."

3051-6

Peelings of potatoes are said to be "strengthening, carrying those influences that are active with the glands of the system."

820-2

These influences or "vital energies" referred to may also be the vitamins, minerals, or both.

"Vegetables," one reading notes, "will build gray matter faster than will meats or sweets.

900-386

Jerusalem artichokes were recommended for a number of individuals with diabetes with the explanation that they carry those properties that have

> an insulin reaction that will produce a cleansing for the kidneys as well as producing the tendency for the reduction of the excess sugar.
>
> 480-39

One individual was also told that these would

> tend to correct those inclinations for the incoordination between the activities of the pancreas as related to the kidney and bladder.
>
> 1523-7

These were never recommended in large amounts, but one about the size of a hen's egg at a time; in some cases once a day, in others once or twice a week, and alternately raw and cooked.

Perhaps the strangest or least understood physiological effect of foods spoken of, and one repeated in many readings, is the effect of eating foods grown in the vicinity where the body resides, rather than those shipped in. This "prepares the system to acclimate itself to any given territory (3542-1). And will more quickly adjust a body to a particular area or climate than any other thing." Further, this is more important than "any specific set of fruit, vegetables . . . or what not."

4047-1

Acid and Alkaline Balance

Readings frequently emphasized the importance of maintaining the correct balance of acid and alkaline reactions in the body through the kinds and combinations of foods taken. Though "an over-alkalinity is much more harmful than a little tendency occasionally for acidity" (808-3), apparently it is much more rare, the emphasis throughout being on more of alkaline-reacting foods.

In response to a question asked concerning common contagious diseases, this answer was given:

If an alkalinity is maintained in the system—especially with the lettuce, carrots, and celery, these in the blood supply will maintain such a condition as to immunize a person.   480-19

Colds are often the result, according to the readings, of an unbalancing of the alkalinity of the system:

Cold cannot—does not exist in alkalines.   808-3

How to maintain the correct balance, "about 20% acid to 80% alkaline-producing," (1523-3), sufficiently alkaline yet not too much so?

The less activities there are in physical exercise or manual activity, the greater should be the alkaline reacting foods taken. Energies or activities may burn acids;—but those who lead the sendentary life or the non-active life can't go on sweets or too much starches . . . these should be well balanced.   798-1

An over-acidity may be produced by overeating of sweets, especially before sufficient food has been taken at meals.

The acidity is produced by taking too much sugar in the system in candies, and in those properties as were taken before the stomach was filled with foods, and then overloading the system at such times (294-86), or by combining sweets and starches (340-32), or several starches at the same meal. 416-18

An abundance of vegetables and fruits, especially citrus fruits, helps to maintain the alkalinity of the system. Lemons especially are a good alkalizer, and the readings consistently recommend adding a little lemon juice, (or lime) to orange juice. (See 2072-3.) Vegetables should be in the proportions of three that grow above the gound to one that grows below the ground, and one leafy vegetable to every one of the pod vegetables.

Sweets and Chocolate

Although warning is frequently given against an excess of sweets in the diet, some are said to be necessary "to form sufficient alcohol for the system" (487-11). Or, as stated in one reading:

the forces in sweets to make for the proper activity through the action of the gastric flows are as necessary as body-building [elements], for these become body-building in making for the proper fermentation (if it may be called so) in the digestive activities. 808-3

The kind of sweets is important, as well as the amounts. Those sweets recommended were grape sugars, beet sugars, raw cane sugars and honey, especially in the honeycomb. Date sugar too is now available, another natural sweetening. One reading recommended:

Chocolates that are plain, not those of any brand that carry corn starches, should be taken—or not those that carry too much of the cane sugar. 487-11

Several later readings, however, warned against chocolates during the war years. Said one, given in 1944, "Chocolate that is prepared in the present is not best for any diet." 4047-1

26

The "Do Not's"

One individual was advised, "then, it is well that the body not become as one that couldn't do this, that or the other; or as a slave to an idea of a set diet (1568-2). Nevertheless, the readings frequently recommended that certain foods and combinations of foods be avoided.

Starches and sweets, except in small amounts, should not be taken at the same meal, nor should there be several starchy foods taken together, since this produces too much acidity in the system. Neither should bread and other starches that grow above the ground be taken with meats. Potatoes, especially the peelings of same, are preferable to breads with meats.

That citrus fruits should not be taken with cereals was a consistent warning. One reading gave this explanation:

for this changes the acidity of the stomach to a detrimental condition. For citrus fruits will act as an eliminant when taken alone, but when taken with cereals they become as weight, rather than as an active force in the gastric forces of the stomach itself.   481-1

Coffee or tea should not be taken with milk or cream, for this is hard on the digestion.   5097-1

From the information given in different readings, apparently the effect of coffee or tea alone varies—for some individuals being harmful, but not for others.

Onions and radishes (raw) should not be taken at the same meal with celery and lettuce, one individual was told, though either might be taken at different times. (See 2732-1.)

Oysters should never be taken with whiskey, as this produces a chemical reaction that is bad for most stomachs.   2583-1

Fried foods should never be eaten, according to the readings, nor vegetables cooked with bacon or fats. Canned foods containing superficial or artificial preservatives should be avoided. Benzoate of soda was specifically mentioned as one of these. Carbonated drinks in most cases were warned against, being referred to as "slop" (5545-2), nor should cane sugar in quantities be used.

Warning is given against using some foods cooked in aluminum, especially where a "disturbed hepatic eliminating force" exists. (1196-7). For this "produces a hardship upon the activities of the kidneys as related to the lower hepatic circulation, or [affects] the uric acid that is a part of the activity of the kidneys in eliminating same from the system" (843-7).

Specifically mentioned were tomatoes, or cabbage:

There are some foods that are affected in their activity by aluminum, especially in the preparation of certain fruits, or tomatoes, or cabbage. But most others it is very well.   1852-1

Many readings recommended that bananas not be eaten, unless, like raw apples, alone, uncombined with other food.

When rabbits are cleaned, "be sure the tendon in both left legs is removed, or that as might cause a fever" (2514-4).

Warnings were repeatedly given against eating pork, except for a little crisp breakfast bacon occasionally. One individual was told of the result, in his or her case, of eating pork:

The character of dross it makes in the body-functioning causes a fungi that produces in the system a crystallization of the muscles and nerves in portions of the body . . . These distresses began as acute pain, rheumatic or neuritis . . . This is pork—the effect of same.   294-41

Red meats, or heavy meats not well cooked, were frequently warned against—while fish, fowl, and lamb were recommended, and wild game, properly prepared, was said to be preferable to other meats. (See 2514-4.)

Meat—To Eat or Not To Eat

Whether an individual should eat meat or abstain has long been a disputed question among health-minded and spiritual-minded individuals. The attitude of the readings on this subject was definite and consistent. One individual was told:

> Meats of certain characters are necessary in the body building forces in this system and should not be wholly abstained from in the present. Spiritualize those influences, those activities, rather than abstaining.
>
> 295-6

Another reading had this to say:

> This, to be sure, is not an attempt to tell the body to go back to eating meat. But do supply, then, through the body forces, supplements, either in vitamins or in substitutes. This is necessary for those who would hold to these [vegetarian] influences . . .

> But purifying of mind is of the mind, not of the body. For, as the Master gave, it is not that which entereth in the body, but that which cometh out, that causes sin. It is what one does with the purpose; for all things are pure in themselves and are for the sustenance of man—body, mind and soul. And remember, these must work together.
>
> 5401-1

Attitudes and Emotions

What importance do attitudes and emotions have in relation to foods? Much, according to the readings. That strong emotions such as anger, fear, or worry have an adverse effect upon the digestive system is well known, and confirmed in the readings to the extent that they advise, "Never when under strain, very tired, very excited or very mad, should the body take foods into the system" (137-30).

But the readings go further concerning the effect of attitude upon the assimilation of food and what mind "as a builder" accomplishes in constructing the body. Thus,

As to what you eat, see it doing what you would have it do.

Now the question is often considered as to why there are different effects under different conditions, from use of vegetable, mineral, or combination compounds. The difference is in the consciousness of the individual body. Give one a dose of clear water, with the impression that it will act as salts—and how often will the water act in that manner. It is the same with impressions to the whole organism. For each cell of the blood stream, each corpuscle, is a whole universe in itself.

One who fills the mind, the very being, with an expectancy of God will see His movement, His manifestation, in the mind and sun, the earth and flowers—the inhabitants of the earth. And so, as the body is built, is the food taken just to gratify an appetite? Or to fulfill a purpose, make it better able to magnify what the body-mind-soul has chosen to stand for?

Thus it will not matter so much what is eaten, or where or when; but just knowing it is consistent with what is desired to be accomplished through the body— that does matter!

As has been given of old—(Daniel 1:5-17). The children of Israel stood with the sons of the heathen, and all ate from the king's table; and that which was taken exercised the imagination of the body in physical desires; strong drink, strong meats, condiments that magnify desires within the body. And these, as Daniel well understood, built not for God's service. He chose, rather, that the everyday common food would be given, so that the body and mind might be a more perfect channel for the manifestations of God. For the Creator's forces are in every force and made manifest in the earth. 341-31

May we, as Daniel, choose that which will build such a temple to serve, magnify, and glorify God!

CHAPTER 3: THE NORMAL DIET

What is a good everyday diet to follow, which will promote good health and keep the individual as a body-mind-spirit *unit* functioning on a high level? We are not born with this knowledge; we must learn it. The Edgar Cayce readings contribute a great deal of information to enlarge our understanding.

For purposes of comparison, let us first consider the *Basic 7* Food Groups which have been established as a guide for a normal daily diet by the Bureau of Human Nutrition and Home Economics, Agricultural Administration of the U.S. Department of Agriculture.

In the leaflet, *National Good Guide,* the *Basic 7* food groups are outlined, and people are advised to eat foods daily from all seven categories. By doing this, we obtain food elements that (1) yield energy; (2) supply materials for growth and upkeep; and (3) keep the body in good running order.

Here is the list of *Basic 7;*

1. Leafy, Green and Yellow Vegetables—One or more servings daily.

2. Citrus Fruit, tomatoes, raw cabbage and other high Vitamin C foods—One or more servings daily.

3. Potatoes and other vegetables and fruit—Two or more servings daily.

4. Milk, Cheese and ice cream:
   Children through teens ages—3 to 4 cups of milk daily.

Adults—2 or more cups of milk daily.
Pregnant woman—At least 1 quart of milk daily.
Nursing mother—About 1-1/2 quarts of milk daily.

5. Meat, Poultry, Fish—One serving daily.
Eggs—4 or more a week.
Dried beans, peas, nuts; peanut butter—2 or more servings a week.

6. Bread, flour, cereals—whole-grain enriched or restored—every day.

7. Butter and fortified margarine—some daily.

The Edgar Cayce readings do not of course classify foods into such a *Basic 7* scheme, yet they do agree with the ideal of variety and balance in daily food elements needed. The readings emphasize certain ideas in regard to daily food selections, from whch we might put together these seven points:

1. Eat more fruits and vegetables

2. Watch the Acid-Alkaline balance in the body

3. Avoid certain food combinations

4. Keep a balance between foods grown above and below ground

5. Eat lightly of heavy meats; use fish, fowl and lamb plus eggs and milk

6. Use whole-grain cereals and such products exclusively

7. Avoid fried foods; use fat sparingly

Before citing extracts from the readings to illustrate the above points and compare with the *Basic 7*, we wish to have the reader realize that each reading covered a wide scope. Thus there is a "spillover" of subject matter which is interesting for correlation, and more helpful than if points were isolated.

The reading placed the greatest emphasis upon foods in the first three categories of the *Basic 7:* fruits and leafy, green, yellow, tomatoes, citrus fruits, etc.

Do include often in the diet raw vegetables, prepared in various ways, not merely as a salad, but scraped or grated and combined with gelatin.　　　　　3445-P-1

Often have raw vegetables such as celery, lettuce, carrots and watercress. Prepare these often with gelatin. Do not throw away the juices when grating or preparing any of these, but include the juices in the gelatin, to obtain a greater amount of necessary vitamins.　　　3413-P-1

Eat plenty of raw as well as cooked carrots. Have plenty of lettuce, and tomatoes in moderation—also raw cabbage occasionally. . . . Do not eat too much potatoes, but more of the skins. Eat plenty of onions, raw as well as cooked; and plenty of the legumes such as peas and beans.　　　　　480-P-47

Eat more vegetables! The leafy variety would be preferable to those of the pod nature such as dried beans or peas, or the like.　　　　　1657-P-1

The Acid-Alkaline Balance

The readings recognized the fact that a normal diet may vary with individuals. Some are more active than others. In adjusting the diet to greater or less activity, it is very important to consider striking a balance between foods that produce acid and foods that produce alkaline. Most vegetables are alkaline-reacting; so are most fruits except prunes and cranberries. The readings give the ideal balance, as follows:

Question: What should the diet be?

Answer: It should consist of those foods which will not create too much of an acid nor too much of an alkaline condition throughout the system. It would be better (for this body) to have more of the alkaline-producing than of the acid-producing foods. 140-P-5

In all bodies, the less activity in respect to physical exercise or manual activity, the greater should be the amount of alkaline-reacting foods taken. Energies or activities may burn acids; but those who lead a sedentary or non-active life cannot go on sweets or too many starches. These foods (alkaline and acid-producing) should be carefully balanced. 798-P-1

Question: What foods are acid-forming for this body?

Answer: All of those that combine fats with sugars. Starches naturally incline toward an acid reaction. But a normal diet is about 20 percent of acid-producing foods to 80 percent of alkaline-producing. 1523-P-3

Have a percentage of 80 percent alkaline-producing to 20 percent acid-producing foods in the diet. It is well, however, that the body not become as one who can't ever do this, that or the other—or as a slave to an idea of a set diet! But do not take citrus fruit juices and cereals at the same meal. Do not take milk or cream in coffee or in tea. Do not eat fried foods of any kind. Do not combine white bread, potatoes, spaghetti, or any two foods of such natures, in the same meal. 1458-P

As indicated, keep the tendency toward alkalinity in the diet. This does not mean there should never be any acid-forming foods in the diet—for over-alkalinity is much more harmful than a little tendency toward acidity occasionally. But remember that there are tendencies in this system toward cold and congestion . . . and cold cannot, does not exist in alkalines. 808-P-3

The diet should be more body-building; that is, contain less of the acid foods and more of the alkaline-reacting foods. Milk and all its products should be a portion of the body's diet now; also those food values making for an easy assimilation of iron, silicon, and those elements

or chemicals found in all kinds of berries, almost all
kinds of vegetables that grow under the ground, almost
all of the vegetables of a leafy nature. Fruits and
vegetables, nuts and the like should form a greater part
of the regular diet in the present . . . Keep closer to the
alkaline diet; using fruits, berries and vegetables
—particularly those carrying iron, silicon, phosphorus
and the like.   480-P-17

In an alkaline system there is less effect of cold and congestion.   270

Food Combinations

On the question of food combinations as such—some good,
some bad—we come to a debatable or controversial point in
respect to opinions held by authorities in the nutrition field.
Medical and scientific opinion at the present time seems to be
divided: some authorities scoff, others are violently *pro*. The
pendulum appears to swing to and fro in this matter. The
reader will probably recall a number of widely publicized
books on diets for arthritis, etc. which are based primarily on
the use of food combinations.

The Edgar Cayce readings greatly stress the value of some
food combinations, and the harm of others. We believe that as
research proceeds to discover how the human body uses the
foods given it, the basic soundness of the Edgar Cayce approach will be verified.

As we find, there is . . . an unbalancing in the alkalinity
of the system. Not an unbalancing produced by the foods
themselves, but rather by the manner of their combination. For as indicated, starches and sweets should not be
taken at the same meal—or at least, not so much taken
together. That's why it is that ice cream is so much better
for a body than pie which combines starches and
sweets.   340-P-31

*Question: What foods can be used with citrus fruits to
make a complete meal?*

Answer: Any foods that may be eaten at any time, save whole-grain cereals. 2072-P-9

Question: Are a quart of milk a day and orange juice every day helpful?

Answer: Orange juice and milk are helpful, but these should be taken at opposite ends of the day and not together. 274-P-6

Questios: What foods should I avoid?

Answer: It is rather the *combination* of foods that makes for disturbance with most physical bodies, as with this one.

In its office activities in its present surroundings, preferably use those foods which tend toward greater alkaline reaction. Hence avoid combinations where corn, potatoes, rice, spaghetti or the like are all taken at the same meal . . . all of which tend to make for too great a quantity of starch—especially (undesirable) if any meat is taken at such a meal. If no meat is taken, the reaction of these starches is quite different. For the gastric flow in the digestive system is of such kinds that one reaction of the gastric flow is required for starch and another for proteins—and still another for digesting carbohydrates combined with starches of such kinds. In the combinations, then, do not eat great quantities of starch along with proteins or meats. Sweets and meats taken at the same meal are preferable to starches and meats. Of course, small quantities of breads are all right with sweets, but not in large quantities.

Also do not combine acid-reacting fruits with starches other than whole wheat bread! That is: citrus fruits, oranges, apples, grapefuit, limes or lemons—or even tomato juice. And do not have cereals—which contain a greater quantity of starch than most—at the same meal with citrus fruits. 416-B

A comment on the preceding extract is in order, since it is a rule given by most reducing diets not to eat two starches at the same meal. Another reason for not "filling up with starches" is of course that we should not crowd out of the meal the leafy green and yellow vegetables and fruits which we need. The normal diet is thus one which nourishes the body properly but does not overbalance it towards overweight or underweight.

On the subject of food combinations, here is an idea which is probably new to those working in the science of modern dietetics and food research. At least, we believe so for we have never seen any allusion to it. It is that lemon or lime juice be added to other citrus fruit juices.

> It will be much better if you add a little lime juice to the orange juice, and a little lemon juice to the grapefruit juice. Not too much, but a little. It will be much better and act much better with the body. For many of these are hybrids, you see. 3525-P-1

> When orange juice is taken, add lime or lemon juice to it: four parts orange juice to one part lime or lemon.
> 3823-P-2

> Take plenty of citrus fruit juices. . . . With the orange juice, put a little lemon juice—that is, for a glass of orange juice put about two squeezes from a good lemon . . . so that there is up to a half teaspoonful of lemon juice added. And with grapefruit juice, put a little lime juice—about eight to ten drops. Stir these together well before taking, of course. 2072-P-2

> Take whole grain cereals or citrus fruits juices, though not at the same meal. When using orange juice, combine lime with it. When using grapefruit juice, combine lemon with it—just a little. 1523

Here is another idea involving food combinations which is emphasized in the Edgar Cayce readings but not found elsewhere: a judicious use of vegetables growing above the ground versus those growing below the ground. The readings gave no explanation for this distinction; perhaps no one asked for it. At any rate, it seems to be an important point to be considered for normal diets as well as diets recommended in the readings for various bodily ailments.

A normal diet . . . use at least three vegetables that grow above the ground to one that grows under the ground.
3373-P-1

Have at least one meal each day that includes a quantity of raw vegetables such as cabbage, lettuce, celery, carrots, onions and the like. Tomatoes may be used in their season. Do have plenty of vegetables grown above the ground—at least three of these to one grown below the ground. Have at least one leafy vegetable to every one of the pod vegetables taken.
2602-P-1

MEATS

Whether or not to eat meat was one of the questions often asked in the question period of a reading. The answers showed insight into the purposes and ideals of the questioners; at the same time pointing out the need of the body for protein.

This, to be sure, is not an attempt to tell the body to go back to eating meat. But then do supply to the body forces either vitamin supplements or meat substitutes. This is necessary for those who hold to vegetarian influences. . . . But purifying of the mind is *of the mind*, not *of the body*. For as the Master gave, it is not that which entereth into the body but that which cometh out that causes sin. It is what one does with the purpose that matters. For all things are pure in themselves and are for the sustenance of man—for his body, mind and soul. Remember, these must be allowed to work together. . .
5401-P-1

Question: Should the body abstain from meats for its best spiritual development?

Answer: Meats of certain kinds are necessary for the body-building forces in this system and should not be

39

wholly abstained from in the present. Spiritualize those influences and those activities, rather than abstaining from meat. For as He gave, that which cometh out, rather than that which goeth in, defileth the spiritual body.   295-P-6

Scientific opinion is definitely in favor of eating meat for body-building, repair and maintenance of repair functions; and to obtain vitamins, especially vitamin B; for minerals, especially phosphorus and iron; and for the important amino acids which are now being intensively investigated and fitted into the dietary pattern.

Meat is a "complete protein" as are poultry, fish and eggs mentioned in No. 5 of the *Basic 7* food divisions. A "complete protein" is one that contains all the *essential* amino acids (needed by the body to manufacture others) in quantities readily usable by the body.

The Edgar Cayce readings stress the use of meat in moderation, especially certain kinds of meat; also fish and fowl.

Question: Please outline the proper diet, suggesting things to avoid.

Answer: Avoid too many heavy meats, not well cooked. Eat plenty of vegetables of all kinds. Meats taken should preferably be fish, fowl and lamb; others not so often. Breakfast bacon, crisp, may be taken occasionally.
                                                      1710-P-3

Keep away from red meats, ham, or rare steaks or roasts. Rather use fish, fowl and lamb.   3596-P-1

Question: What should the diet be for this body?

Answer: Not too much of meats of any kind. Rather take fowl or fish, and vegetables that clarify the blood. These would be cooked onions, beets, carrots, salsify, raw carrots, celery or lettuce. These will act well with the mental and spiritual forces in the body.   288-P-4

And in the matter of diet, keep away from too much grease or too much of any foods cooked in quantities of grease—whether of hog, sheep, beef or fowl! Rather use the lean protions and those meats which will make for body-building forces throughout. Fish and fowl are the preferred meats. No raw meat, and very little *ever* of hog meat—only bacon. Do not use bacon or fats in cooking the vegetables.   303-P-7

Use plenty of fowl, but prepared in such a way that more of the bone structure itself is used . . . in its reaction through the system; so that assimilation of calcium is obtained. Chew chicken necks, then! Chew the bones of the thigh! Also have the marrow of beef or such as a part of the diet, and eat foods such as vegetables soups rich in the beef which carries the bone marrow . . . and eat the marrow!   1523-P-6

In the diet, keep away from heavy foods. Use those which are body-building; such as beef juice, beef broth, liver, fish, lamb. All of these may be taken but never fried foods.   5269-P-1

Surprisingly, we find high praise in the readings for wild game which is seldom mentioned in tables of nutritional values. The readings caution about preparing rabbit or hare:

Question: Is it all right for me to eat rabbit and squirrel, baked or stewed?

Answer: Any wild game is preferable to other meats, if it is prepared properly. In cooking rabbit, be sure that the tendon in both left legs is removed, for this is the part which might cause a fever, being what is called at times "the wolf" in the rabbit. Prepared in some ways, this might be excellent for some specific disturbance in a body, but it is never well for it to be eaten in a hare.

In preparing squirrel, of course, the same is not true. When squirrel is stewed or well cooked, it is really preferable for the body; but rabbit is all right if that part indicated is removed.   2514-P-4

Eggs, Cheese and Milk

Eggs and cheese are also "complete proteins" valuable in the diet. According to *USDA Bulletins*, the important nutrients in eggs are: protein, vitamin A (in the yolk), iron, vitamin B-1 and B-2. The readings also have good things to say about eggs and cheese; and eggs were frequently recommended for breakfasts, as will be seen in the *Menu* Section.

Eggs may be taken two or three times a week, and cooked in any manner except fried. · 257-P-15

Some elements in eggs are not found in other foods—particularly sulphur. Egg whites cause other elements in the diet to be bad; yet we would take them occasionally. Do not necessarily eat meat if you are that-minded. But remember, it is not what goes in the mouth but what comes out of the mouth that defiles the body. 5399

Take in food values those foods which carry iron and silicon, such as beets, celery and radishes. These cleanse the system. Eat spinach and eggs. . . . Do not eat too heavily of meats except fish, fowl or game. Never use fried meats of any kind for this body, but rather broiled, boiled or baked—and not with much grease. Eat olives of every kind. Cheese and cream are good for this system. 257-P-7

Most of us know—or should know—the importance of drinking enough milk every day. Nutritionists of the United States Department of Agriculture recommend drinking at least 3 cups or 1-1/2 pints of milk a day, for the population as a whole. According to these nutritionists, the national average is less than a pint of milk a day, taken in fluid form. They say that regardless of age, the calcium in milk and dairy products is vital for good health.

The readings recommended milk as a beverage for meals, as will be seen in the *Menu* Section, and gave milk as a source of calcium for those who needed more calcium in the diet. In addition, we have these sidelights on the value of milk:

Irradiated or dried milk, as a rule, is much more healthful for most individuals than raw milk.   480-P-39

Milk in all its forms, and the products of milk, should be a portion of the diet.   903-P-14

It would be well for the general strength to be built up with beef juices, egg and milk drinks, and easily assimilated foods.   265-P-7

Question: Is buttermilk good?

Answer: This depends upon the way in which it is made. If it is the ordinary kind, it would tend to produce gas; but that made by the use of the Bulgarian tablets is good in moderation. Not too much!   404-P-5

Milk and milk products, and leafy green vegetables are rich in calcium and contain little starch.   382-P-6

Whole-Grain Cereals

As the next point in our parallel study of the *Basic 7* we come to #6: *Bread* flour, cereals—"whole-grain, enriched or restored". The readings advocated only whole-grain cereals, used for breakfast or made into bread. In the *Menu* Section of this book, we find several mentions of buckwheat cakes and whole grain cereals prepared for breakfast, as well as whole wheat toast (Readings No. 1523-P-9; 3224-P-2 and 3823-P-2). In Section 4, under Vitamins and Minerals, will also be found references to food values found in cereals and breads. The two extracts given below may be considered merely an introduction to this whole body of information detailed elsewhere.

Rolled or cracked-whole-wheat that is not cooked so long as to destroy the whole vitamin force—this will add to the body the proper portions of iron, silicon and vitamins necessary for building up the blood supply which makes for resistance in the system . . .   840-P-1

Question: What is particularly wrong with my diet?

Answer: The tendency for eating too much starch, pastries, white bread. These should be almost entirely eliminated. Not that you shouldn't eat ice cream, but don't eat cake too! White potatoes, such foods as macaroni or the like, with cheese—eliminate these. They are not very good for the body of this individual, in any form.   416-MS-4

It sounds to us as if No. 416 were worried about over-weight. Certainly the advice given him is good from a dietetic standpoint. Starches and sweets not burnt up by activities are deposited as fat. Yet the Cayce emphasis is not upon obesity as such; but upon keeping the body healthy that it may be a fit temple. The Laws of Balance and Moderation hold true here as in all other aspects of living.

Sweets

Some of us have more of a "sweet tooth" than others. The readings recognized the fact that we have a desire for sweets, and gave this advice:

Question: Please suggest the best sugar for this body.

Answer: Beet sugars are the best for everyone; or cane sugars that are not clarified.   1131-P-2

Keep away from too much sweets, though honey may be taken.   3053-P-3

Keep the body from too much sweets, though have sufficient . . . to form enough alcohol for the system. That is: watch the *kind* of sweets, rather than just taking sweets. Grape sugars would be good—hence grape jellies or sweets of that nature.　　　　　　　　　　487-P-7

Do be careful that there are not quantities of pastries, pies or candies taken; especially chocolates and carbonated-water drinks. These sweets, we find, will be hard on the body.　　　　　　　　　　5218-P-1

Saccharin may be used. Brown sugar is not harmful. Best of all would be to use beet sugar for sweetening. 307-P-3

Question: What type of sweets may be eaten by the body?

Answer: Honey, especially in the honeycomb; or preserves made with beet sugar rather than cane sugar. Not too great a quantity of any of these . . . but enough so that the forces in sweets make for proper activity through the action of gastric flows. . . . For these [sweets] become body-building by producing proper fermentation [if it may be so called] in the digestive activity. Hence two or three times a week, honey used on bread . . . would furnish that activity necessary in the whole system.　　　　　　　　　　808-P-3

Energies or activities may burn acids but those who lead a sedentary or non-active life can't go on sweets or too much starchy food. Yet these should be well-balanced.
　　　　　　　　　　798-P-1

The diet also should be considered. There shouldn't be an excess of acids or sweets—or even an excess of alkalinity. . . . There should be maintained a normal, well-balanced diet that has been proved right for the individual body.　　　　　　　　　　902-1

We come finally to point 7 of the *Basic 7*, butter and fortified margarine. The modern trend in dietetics is away from the use of much fat in the diet. The Edgar Cayce readings

(1901 through 1944) de-emphasized the use of fat throughout all items of the diet. Meats were not to be fried; vegetables were not to be cooked with fat meats; the lean portions of meats instead of the fat portions were nearly always suggested; and butter was mentioned as a light seasoning, along with salt, for vegetables.

CHAPTER 4: FRUITS AND VEGETABLES

"Balance" seems to be a key word in the Cayce readings. We should strive to keep a balance of activities, attitudes, and additionally the chemical composition or balance of our bodies. One of the most important of these physical (or chemical) balances is that of acidity and alkalinity. (See Chapter 1)

Bernard Jensen, D.C., N.D., author, lecturer and Director of Hidden Valley Health Ranch at Escondido, California, is in complete agreement with the Cayce readings, both as to the importance of maintaining this balance and the proportions of different types of foods necessary to do so—that is, 80% alkaline-producing and 20% acid-producing. The correct proportions would be four vegetables and two fruits to one protein and one starch, he says, though he does not recommend keeping these exact proportions each day, but rather approximating them over a period of time.

Dr. Jensen relates two experiments which were performed in relation to the effect of low acidity of the body. In one, turpentine was injected into the leg of a rabbit while it was alkalinized, with very slight damage resulting to the leg. The same amount of turpentine injected into the leg when the rabbit was acidized, however, resulted in inflammation, tissue sloughing and death. In the other experiment it was discovered that among a number of scarlet fever patients two-thirds of those with high acidity developed nephritis, though this complication occurred in only 3% of the cases in which the acidity was low.

When citrus fruits (which are strongly alkaline-producing cause distress, Dr. Jensen states, it may be due to their tendency to stir up acids already accumulated in the body, giving the mistaken impression that they are having a bad effect. ("Vital Foods for Total Health"—Dr. Bernard Jensen Enterprises, Los Angeles, California).

In general, starchy foods, fatty foods, sugar, (either white or raw) and proteins are acid-forming, while fruits and vegetables are alkaline-forming (with a few exceptions). Also, as Dr. Jensen points out, vegetables which are alkaline-forming when fresh may become acid-forming within a few days after being picked. Incorrect combinations of foods, according to the readings, become a factor in producing an over-acid condition.

Alkaline Forming Foods

ALL FRUITS, Fresh and Dried, *except* large Prunes, Plums and Cranberries.

Apples	Grapefruit	Peaches
Apricots	Honey	Pears
Berries	Lemons	Pineapples
Dates	Limes	Raisins
Figs (unsulphured)	Oranges	Small Prunes

ALL VEGETABLES, Fresh and Dehydrated; *except* Legumes, (Dried Peas, Beans and Lentils) and Rhubarb.

Asparagus	Green Peas	Radishes
Beets	Kohlrabi	Rutabaga
Cabbage	Lettuce	Spinach
Carob	Mushrooms	Sprouts
Carrots	Olives (ripe)	String Beans
Cauliflower	Onions	Sweet Potatoes
Celery	Oyster Plant	Tomatoes
Egg Plant	Parsnips	Turnips

MILK
All forms; Buttermilk, Clabber, Sour Milk, Cottage Cheese, Cheese.

Acid Forming Foods

ANIMAL FATS & VEGETABLE OILS
Large Prunes, Plums, Cranberries, Rhubarb.
ALL CEREAL GRAINS
And other such products, as, Bread, Breakfast Foods, etc.,

48

Rolled Oats, Corn Flakes, Corn Meal Mush, Polished Rice, etc. (Brown Rice is less acid forming).

ALL HIGH STARCH AND PROTEIN FOODS—White Sugar, Syrups made from White Sugar. (Starchy foods in combination with fruits or proteins are acid combinations and should be avoided.)

NUTS

Peanuts, English Walnuts, Pecans, Filberts, Coconut.

LEGUMES

Dried Beans, Dried Peas, Lentils.

MEATS

Beef, Pork, Lamb, Veal.

POULTRY

Chicken, Turkey, Duck, Goose, Guinea Hen, Game.

VISCERAL MEATS

Heart, Brains, Kidney, Liver, Sweetbreads, Thymus.

EGG WHITES

(Yolks are not acid forming.)

Tables of Alkaline Forming Foods and Acid Forming Foods—See Continental Scale Works booklet, "Scientific Weight Control," edited by Dr. James M. Booher, M.D.

Fruits

Fresh ripe fruits may be served raw in a variety of combinations as salads and juices, and are so satisfyingly delicious "as is" that except for apples there seems little reason for cooking them. Raw apples were often advised against in the readings, and never, to our knowledge, recommended as part of the regular diet, other than in "the Apple Diet":

3 days of raw apples only, and then olive oil (1/2 cup), and we will cleanse all toxic forces from any system.

820-2

Fully ripe fruits, especially when ripened on the tree or vine, have a greater vitamin content as well as better flavor. In order to preserve the nutritive value they should be chilled as soon as ripened and picked, handled carefully to avoid bruising,—washed quickly and peeled or cut just before using. Berries should be washed before being stemmed, rather than after, but should not be washed before storing, as they bruise

49

easily. If it is unavoidable that fruits should stand for some time after being peeled or cut, discoloration and vitamin loss may be lessened by having them chilled before peeling, by mixing cut fruit with a little lemon juice to retard enzyme activity—returning them to the refrigerator as quickly as possible. The same precautions apply to the squeezing of orange juice—the juice should be extracted just before being used, but there is less loss of vitamin C if the oranges are chilled before being squeezed, and the juice kept refrigerated with air excluded.

Stewed Dried Fruit

Dried fruits should be washed quickly and if soaked, cooked in the water used for soaking. They may be cooked without soaking, or may be tenderized by soaking in hot (boiling) water with no further cooking, but with either method, the water or juice should not be disturbed, as it will contain much nutritive value.

Method #1 - Cover fruit with water and bring to a boil. Remove from heat and allow to stand overnight.

Method #2 - Bring 2 cups of water to a boil. Add 1 pound of fruit (dried), cover utensil, reduce heat and simmer until fruit is tender (about 12 to 15 minutes).

Dried fruits contain a large proportion of sugar and usually require no added sweetening. For variety, bits of lemon or orange rind may be added to prunes, apples, pears or figs during cooking, or small amounts of cloves and cassia buds, or stick cinnamon to prunes, pears, peaches or apples.

Stewed dried fruits may be served with cereal, or sprinkled with ground nuts or grated coconut, or served with cream as a breakfast dish or healthful dessert; stewed or raw dried fruits may be used in cakes, cookies, confections and puddings. For the latter, see the chapter on Desserts & Sweets.

Baked Apricots

1/2 pound dried apricots	1/2 cup honey
1 cup seeded raisins	Juice of 1 lemon
2 cups water	1 orange

Wash apricots, add raisins and water and place in baking dish. Cover and bake at 325° for 2-1/2 hrs. Remove from oven, add honey and lemon juice, stir and chill. Before serving, top with sliced peeled orange.

MUMMY FOOD

For those not familiar with the origin of the recipe for "Mummy Food"—Edgar Cayce had a dream (December 2, 1937) concerning the discovery of ancient records in Egypt in which a mummy came to life and helped to translate these records. The mummy, he dreamed, gave directions for the preparation of a food which she required. (See 294-189 Supplement.) Thus the name, "mummy food."

Other readings for particular individuals recommended this same combination. One such was as follows:

> and for this especial body, a mixture of dates and figs that are dried, cooked with a little corn meal—a very little sprinkled in—then this taken with milk, should be almost a spiritual food for the body.   275-46

More detailed instructions were:

> . . . Equal portions of black figs or Assyrian figs and Assyrian dates—these ground together or cut very fine, and to a pint of such a combination put half a handful of corn meal or crushed wheat. These cooked together.
>
> 274-46

"Half a handful" is, of course, a rather indefinite amount and the amount of water is not given. The following has been tried and found satisfactory:

Mummy Food

| 1/2 cup chopped pitted dates | 1 to 1-1/2 cups water |
| 1/2 cup chopped dried black figs | 1 rounded tbsp. corn meal |

Cook over low heat, stirring frequently, for ten minutes or longer. Serve with milk or cream. Serves 2 to 4.

Baked Apples

Wash and core large red or yellow apples, one for each person to be served. Set in baking dish and stuff center of each with a mixture of chopped raisins and nuts. Honey may be added to this mixture if desired. Sprinkle with cinnamon, nutmeg, or grated lemon rind. Put piece of butter on top and add 1/4 cup boiling water. Cover and bake in hot oven until tender; 20 min. or longer, depending on variety of apples.

Serve hot or cold, with top milk, cream or yogurt.

Baked Pears

| 4 medium sized pears | 1/4 cup honey |
| 1/4 cup boiling water | 1 tbsp. lemon juice |

Scrub pears, remove blossom end and put stem side up in baking dish. Mix honey, boiling water and lemon juice and pour around pears. Add 2 tsp. butter if desired. Cover and bake at 375° for 1 hr., basting occasionally.

If large pears are used they may be cut in half, lengthwise, the cut surface brushed with lemon juice, then cooked as above.

Baked Peaches

Cut unpeeled, scrubbed peaches in half and remove seed. Place in baking dish, pour 1/4 cup water around them. In center of each peach half put 1 tsp. or more of honey, top with a small chunk of butter, sprinkle lightly with cinnamon or cloves. Cover and bake at 350° to 375° just until tender.

Baked Bananas

Place peeled bananas in shallow baking dish, sprinkle with lemon juice, and add 1 tsp. honey for each banana if desired. Bake 10 to 15 min. at 375°.

Apple Sauce

Bring to boil 1/2 cup water in saucepan. Drop in 2 lbs. of cooking apples, washed and quartered but not peeled or cored. Cover, reduce heat and steam until soft, about 15 min. Press apples through a collander or food mill, chill, and sweeten to taste with raw sugar or honey. Flavor if desired with cinnamon, nutmeg, or grated lemon or orange rind.

Stewed Whole Apples

Peel washed and cored apple 1/4 of the way down and put peeled side down in saucepan containing 1/2 cup boiling water. Cover, boil for 1 min. then reduce heat and simmer until tender when tested with a toothpick. Turn peeled side up, sprinkle with raw sugar and cinnamon or nutmeg and top with butter. Brown under broiler.

APPETIZERS

Orange-Apricot:

Combine in each serving glass
2/3 cup orange juice   1/3 cup apricot juice or thin
                                           purée

Stir, garnish with sprig of fresh mint. Serve cold.

Black Raspberry-Peach:

Mix directly in each serving glass
1/3 cup black raspberries   1/3 cup unsweetened
1/3 cup diced yellow peaches   pineapple juice

Set in refrigerator until time to serve.

Pear-Persimmon:

1 medium-size fresh pear,   1-1/3 cups pineapple or
   washed, unpeeled   grapefruit juice
2 large unpeeled California
   persimmons

Dice pear and soak in juice for 1/2 hr. Have persimmons frozen solid and just before serving cut them in small cubes and combine with pears and juice.

Decorative Juice Cubes

Use any clear light-colored juice. Half fill ice cube trays with juice and set into freezing compartment until ice crystals form over top. Quickly arrange small fresh rasperries, strawberries, or bits of orange or lemon peel with small mint leaves, to simulate flower arrangement, in center of each cube. Freeze until solid, then add enough juice to fill the tray and complete freezing. Add these cubes to glasses of chilled juice just before serving.

Frozen Fruit Purées

Beat or mash through collander or food mill, soft stewed apricots, plums, peaches, or other fruit. Add honey to taste. Freeze in freezing compartment, stirring or beating 2 or 3 times. May be served in sherbet glasses with meat course or as dessert, or stored in freezer in plastic containers for use when fresh fruit is not available.

Fruit Aspics

Combine in saucepan 1/2 cup fruit juice and 1 tbsp. gelatin, and soak for 5 min. Heat slowly until gelatin is dissolved and add 1-1/2 cups fruit purée. Add 1 or 2 tbsp. lemon juice if purée is not tart. Pour into mold, chill until firm. Unmold and serve with meat.

Sunny Compote

In a covered dish, slice bananas and plump moist figs. Mix together, then sprinkle chopped sunflower seeds over them. Keep the dish covered until time to serve.

Berry Bowl

1 cup fresh strawberries	1 cup black raspberries
1 cup raw blueberries	1 cup black cherries

Blend fruits in a bowl and keep covered until time for serving. Add honey and nuts or sunflower seeds if desired.

Raw Winter Pears

Pare, core and slice winter pears into a serving dish. Dribble with honey or maple syrup and season with 1/4 tsp. of ginger. Cover until time to serve.

Apricot Conserve

Pit and mash fresh apricots. Stir in the desired amount of honey and thicken with blanched ground almonds.

Strawberry Sherbet

1 pkg. Polar frosted
   strawberries

1 cup orange juice
1 cup water

Mash strawberries, add orange juice and water. Pour into refrigerator tray and freeze. Serve with heavy whipped cream.

Fresh Peach Mousse

5 peaches, mashed
1/2 pint whipped cream

2 tbsp. maple syrup
1/3 cup almonds, ground

Mash fine either fresh peaches or soaked dried peaches, and chill. Then combine with whipped cream. Add maple syrup and nuts. Chill before serving.

Banana Delight

Stem 2 cups dried figs. Chop fine and put in covered dish, cover with hot water. Cover and let stand over night or several hours. Then mash fine. Slice 4 bananas in a casserole-type dish, pour the mashed figs over them. Sprinkle with chopped English walnuts or peanuts. Keep covered, unchilled, until serving time.

VEGETABLES

If eighty percent of our food is to be alkaline-producing, as recommended, probably at least fifty percent will be in the form of vegetables. Certainly it is worth while to use considerable care in their selection and preparation.

Vegetables should be freshly gathered if possible. Frozen vegetables, however, are preferable to those which have been several days in shipment, or to commercially canned foods which have added chemical preservatives.

Bright yellow and intensely green vegetables provide the greatest concentration of minerals and vitamins. Green leafy vegetables also contain an anti-stress factor as yet unidentified[1]: perhaps this is why the readings advised at least one leafy vegetable with each one of the pod variety.

Nutritive value may be lost by peeling, since most of the minerals are concentrated just under the skin; by boiling, which leaches out the minerals, sugars, and water-soluble vitamins; and by destruction of vitamins through the action of enzymes in the presence of oxygen and light.

Vegetables, except for potatoes and dry onions, should be washed, dried and returned to the refrigerator, and then when cooked, heated rapidly, as enzymes are inactive when cold and are killed by heat. Having the cooking utensils heated and filled with steam, plus leaving the lid on during cooking are important, as vitamin B is destroyed by heating in the presence of light. Alkali destroys vitamin C; thus, soda should never be used in cooking vegetables. Minerals in hard water are another offender in this respect. Contact with copper or iron also destroys vitamin C and should be carefully avoided.

Cooking vegetables by the steam pressure method helps to retain the vitamins, so the readings point out (462-14), but care must be taken to avoid over-cooking when using this method. Cooking time should be checked precisely and the utensil cooled immediately when cooking time has expired. Cooking in Patapar paper (trade name of Paterson Parchment Co., Bristol, Pa.) was recommended. (1196-6) Note: Cooking parchment, available in most Health Food stores, also meets the requirement for preserving nutrients, retaining the juices of the vegetable which contain the vitamins and minerals, and excluding oxygen and light. The paper should be tied tightly around the vegetable to eliminate dead air space, and put into rapidly boiling water. Time-tables must be relied on to indicate when sufficiently cooked.

[1] "Let's Get Well," by Adelle Davis.

Timetable for Steaming Vegetables

	Minutes		Minutes
Artichokes, Globe	20-30	Kale	8-10
Artichokes, Jerusalem	6-10	Kohlrabi	9-10
Asparagus	10-15	Leek, sliced	8-10
Beans, Green or Wax	15-20	Mushrooms, chopped	8-10
Beans, fresh Limas	15-20	Mustard Greens, shredded	5-8
Beets, whole small	30-35	Okra	5-8
Beets, grated	5-8	Onions, sliced	5-8
Beet Leaves	3-5	Onions, whole	20-25
Broccoli	8-10	Parsley	5
Brussels Sprouts	10-12	Parsnips, sliced	10-15
Cabbage, Chinese	4-7	Parsnips, whole	20
Cabbage, quartered	4-7	Peas, fresh Green	8-10
Cabbage, shredded	3	Peppers, Green	8-10
Carrots, small whole	20-25	Potatoes, halved Sweet	30-35
Carrots, grated	5-8	Potatoes, halved White	30-35
Cauliflower, in pieces	8-10	Rutabagas, cubed	25-30
Celery	8-10	Spinach	3-5
Celery root	20-25	Squash, Summer	8-10
Corn, fresh	3-5	Swiss Chard	8
Dandelion Greens	3-5	Turnips	20-25
Endive	3-5	Turnip Greens, shredded	5
Eggplant, cubed	8-10	Tomatoes	3-5
Garbanzo Peas	180		

Lemon Broccoli

1-1/2 lbs. broccoli   2 tbsp. honey
1 tbsp. lemon juice

Trim outer leaves and tough ends of broccoli, split any thick
stalks, then cut stalks and flowerets into about 3 in. lengths.

Steam, covered, in a small amount of salted water in a medium size saucepan, 10 min., or just until crisply tender.
Drain carefully, retaining water, and spoon into heated serving bowl. Mix lemon juice, water drained from broccoli, and
honey, and drizzle over broccoli.

Steamed Celery Cabbage

1 medium size head Chinese   1 tsp. celery seeds
   cabbage   1 tsp. salt

Shred cabbage fine, wash well and drain. Place in a large
frying pan (no need to add any water), sprinkle with salt and
celery seeds, and cover. Steam 3 min. or just until crisply tender. Serve with cooking juices.

Asparagus with Citrus Sauce

1-1/2 lbs. asparagus, steamed   4 tbsp. orange juice
2 tbsp. butter   Grated rind of 1/2 orange
2 egg yolks, well beaten   1/4 tsp. paprika
1 tbsp. lemon juice   Dash of salt

Set steamed asparagus aside. To make sauce: combine butter,
salt, egg yolks, paprika and grated orange rind. Cook over hot
water, stirring constantly until thick and smooth. Add orange
and lemon juice and beat until smooth. Serve over asparagus.

59

Sliced Baked Beets

8 small beets, sliced	1-1/2 tbsp. butter
1 tbsp. honey	1-1/2 tsp. lemon juice
3/8 tsp. salt	2-1/2 tbsp. water
1/8 tsp. nutmeg	1 small onion, chopped

Place beets in layers in greased baking dish. Season with honey, salt and nutmeg. Dot with butter, add lemon juice, water and onions. Bake in moderate oven 30 min. or until tender. Sprinkle with parsley and serve. Serves 4-5.

Note: for those who object to onions, substituting celery wherever recipes call for onions has been found altogether satisfactory.

Baked Acorn Squash with Pineapple

3 acorn squash, halved	4 tbsp. butter
1/2 cup crushed pineapple, unsweetened, drained	1/4 tsp. ground nutmeg
	1 tsp. salt
2 tbsp. honey	4 tbsp. butter

Place cleaned and halved squash in greased baking dish and divide honey and butter mixture into center of each half. Cover and bake at 400° for 30 min. or until tender. Scoop cooked squash out of shells leaving about 1/4 in. remaining in shells. Mash squash and combine with 4 tbsp. butter and remaining ingredients that have been heated until well blended. Spoon back into shells and return to hot oven for 15 min.

Baked Carrots

Mix 1 lb. coarsely shredded carrots with 1/4 cup minced onions, 1/4 cup water, 2 tbsp. butter, 1-1/4 tsp. salt, 1/4 tsp. celery salt. Bake covered at 375° for 45 min. or until tender.

Green Peas with Celery and Ripe Olives

2 cups celery, sliced at angle
    into 2-in. pieces
2 tbsp. vegetable oil
2 pkgs. frozen peas, partly
    thawed

20 pitted ripe olives, halved
1/2 tsp. salt
1/4 tsp. pepper

Use large frying pan, on low heat. Stir celery in oil thoroughly until all cut surfaces are coated. Cover and cook celery in oil for 10 min., shaking occasionally; add peas, cover and continue cooking at same temperature for 6 min., shaking several times. Add 1 tbsp. water if necessary during cooking. Stir in olives, salt and pepper. Serves 6-8.

Raw Carrots and Peas

2 cups raw peas

2 cups raw baby carrots

Top and wash baby carrots. Cut them into chunks not much larger than the peas and put both in a covered dish. Serve raw. Neither dressing nor seasoning is needed. They are delicious "as is."

Garbanzos Creole

2 cups cooked garbanzos
1/2 Spanish onion, chopped

1 cup home-canned tomatoes

Simmer these ingredients together until the onion is tender. Serve hot. 1/4 tsp. honey may be added, if desired.

Succotash

Open one package each of frozen sweet corn and green lima beans (or home-canned ones) and simmer together gently, seasoning with sea kelp, dried marjoram and 1 tbsp. of salad oil. Add a shake of black pepper and garnish with green peppers cut in fancy shapes. Serve hot in a heavy utensil.

Young Beets and Greens

Wash and cook young beets gently until tender, probably 10 min. Cut the little beets off the tops and skin them. Chop the beet tops and place in a serving dish, with the baby beets nested in the center. Dress with oil, vinegar and honey and a faint dusting of cinnamon.

Jerusalem Artichokes

Jerusalem artichokes, frequently recommended in the readings for individuals with diabetes or a tendency to same, were also said to

"produce a cleansing for the kidneys" (480-39), and to "correct those inclinations for the incoordination between the activities of the pancreas as related to the kidneys and bladder" (1523-7).

There is no indication whether they are advisable in the normal diet, but they have been used by many as a vegetable rather than as a medicine with no apparent negative effects.

The Jerusalem artichoke has been referred to as the "starchless potato." It is a nutty-flavored tuber containing unulin (not insulin) and levulose, and good amounts of potassium and thiamine. They are good steamed (in Patapar paper, the readings advised) or raw, in salads, grated or thinly sliced. They are planted like potatoes, says an article in *Prevention Magazine*, yield better than potatoes, and are handled and harvested in the same way, except that they are perennials and should be planted in a permanent place. Also, they will not keep well for any length of time out of the ground, so should be left in the ground, under a heavy mulch, during the winter and dug up as needed. The blossoms, similar to small sunflowers, reach a height of from 6 to 12 feet, so they should be planted in a place where these will not be undesirable.

Seed Sprouts

The section on sprouts is included not because of specific recommendations as such in the readings, but for the fact that they offer an excellent way of obtaining a fresh supply of alkaline-producing vegetables with all the vitamins and minerals.

In many sections of the country it is difficult to obtain fresh salad greens or vegetables during large parts of the year, and impossible in most areas to have them year round, grown ("in the vicinity in which the body resides").

Sprouting seeds increases their vitamin content and changes their starch into a simple sugar, easy to digest. The cooking time of beans, such as navy beans, red beans, etc., which ordinarily require two to three hours may be shortened to 10-15 min. by sprouting, giving the double advantage of saving fuel and avoiding the destruction of food values which takes place during long cooking.

Many different seeds may be used. Almost every kind of bean, especially mung and soy beans, peas, lentils, wheat, rye, oats, corn, barley, millet, alfalfa, clover and parsley are among those which produce tasty and nutritious sprouts.

They may be used as soon as the spout is seen, and the vitamin content continues to increase as the sprout grows. However, many kinds of sprouts become less tasty if allowed to grow too long.

Catharyn Elwood, in her book, "Feel Like a Million," states her preference for the length of the different sprouts thus:

Wheat sprouts—length of the seed.
Mung bean sprouts—1-1/2 to 2 inches
Alfalfa sprouts—1 to 2 inches
Pea and Soy Bean sprouts—good either short or long
Lentil sprouts—1 inch
Sunflower seed sprouts—length of seed.

How to Sprout Seeds

There are several methods of sprouting seeds, some of which seem to work better than others. Probably the more satisfactory method depends on seed size. You may have to experiment to find the method that suits you best, but the principle of all is the same: the seeds must be kept warm and moist, must get enough oxygen, and should be kept in the dark.

#1—Put soy beans in an earthenware pot with the hole in the bottom covered by a piece of crockery. For 1/4 lb. of beans use a 2-qt. pot. Pour water over them and make sure it drains off. Keep beans warm and moist, sprinkling them about twice each day (more often if necessary). The beans may be soaked for about 6 hours, before being placed in the pot.

#2—Wash wheat, soak over night, drain and rinse in the morning, add fresh water and put in a dark place. Repeat draining and rinsing 3 times a day for 3 days. The evening of the 3rd day drain wheat thoroughly, put in a shallow pan in a dark place until morning, when sprouts should be of the proper length.

#3—Place about 1 tablespoon of alfalfa seed in a wide-mouth jar, cover with water; place a piece of nylon stocking or fine nylon net over the mouth of the jar and secure with a rubber band. Let stand over night or eight hours, out of light. When time is complete, drain well, rinse slowly and easily and place jar on its side out of light. At least 3 times a day cover with water and drain again. After each draining, return the jar to its side. If the humidity is low, there is no danger of the seeds drying out. To avoid this, sprinkle them occasionally throughout the day with water. In 3 to 5 days the sprouts will reach a length of 1 to 2 inches and are ready for use. Remove the sprouts from the jar, place in large bowl and rinse carefully to remove the brown hulls, using a collander.

#4—Scatter seed on damp bath towel. Roll towel loosely, sprinkle towel whenever necessary to keep damp. This method may be most successful with small seeds.

When sprouts are of the desired length put in large bowl, wash thoroughly to remove hulls if necessary, and store in refrigerator in crisper or plastic bag.

Using Sprouts

Sprouts may be eaten by themselves with your favorite
seasoning, in sandwiches, salads, or many cooked dishes.
Sprouted wheat may be added to bread dough for an interesting variation. Soy and mung bean sprouts may be served as a
cooked vegetable.

Mushroom Chop Suey

2 tbsp. vegetable oil
3 cups onion, diced
3 cups celery, diced
1 cup beef stock or chicken
broth
1 can mushrooms, broken or
sliced

2 tbsp. soy sauce
2 tsp. Bead molasses
1 tsp. salt
2 tbsp. corn starch
1 lb. mung or soy bean
sprouts

Sauté onion and celery slowly in vegetable oil for a few
minutes, add 3/4 cup stock or broth and simmer for 10 min.,
add mushrooms. Mix remaining broth with corn starch, soy
sauce, Bead molasses and salt. Add to vegetables and cook,
stirring constantly until thickened. Add bean sprouts and simmer 5 min. Serve with cooked brown rice.
Chinese chestnuts and bamboo sprouts may be added if
available. If raw Chinese chestnuts are used, slice thin and
add with sauce.

Chicken-Bean Sprout Chop Suey

1 lb. bean sprouts
1/2 cup onion slices
2 tbsp. butter
2 cups diced chicken or turkey
1 cup celery, diced
1 can water chestnut slices
1/2 cup chicken bouillon or
turkey broth

2 tbsp. arrowroot (corn starch)
1/4 tsp. salt
1/4 cup water
2 tbsp. soy sauce
1/2 cup slivered almonds

Cook onions in butter until tender, but not brown. Add
chicken or turkey, celery, water chestnuts, broth, and heat to

boiling point. Combine arrowroot, seasonings, water and soy sauce. Stir into poultry mixture. Cook until thickened. Add sprouts and nuts. Serves 8.

Egg Foo Yung

2 med. onions	2 tbsp. vegetable oil
3 med. green peppers	1/2 tsp. salt
4 eggs, beaten whole	1 lb. fresh bean sprouts

Chop or cut fine onions and peppers, add other ingredients, and mix well. Spoon onto a hot oiled grill and sauté until light brown on both sides.

Soy Bean Sprout Omelet

1 egg, separated	2 tbsp. soy bean sprouts
1 tbsp. water	1 tsp. butter, sweet
1 tsp. vegetized salt	

Beat egg white until frothy. Add water and salt. Continue beating until stiff, then fold in the well-beaten yolk and the bean sprouts. Pour into a hot, buttered omelet pan and cook over the fire 2 min. Bake in moderate oven, 350°, for 3 min. or until done.

Bean Sprout Omelet

3 eggs	Salt
1 cup bean sprouts, cooked	Radishes to garnish
1/2 cup raw sweet cream	

Beat eggs until light, add bean sprouts, cream and salt. Cook in double boiler until eggs are set. Garnish with thin slices of crisp red radishes.

Mung Bean Sprouts

1 tbsp. butter   2 cups mung bean sprouts
1/2 cup onion, chopped

Sauté chopped onion in a pan. Remove from heat and add mung beans. Shake or carefully stir the mixture until sprouts are well covered.

Alfalfa Sprouts Rarebit

Put the following ingredients in blender and blend well:

2 cups water   1 tsp. onion powder
3 tbsp. raw cashews   3 tbsp. arrowroot powder
1 tsp. salt
1 tbsp. whole wheat pastry
   flour

Pour liquid into pan, on low heat, and stir constantly until sauce thickens. Remove from fire and add the following ingredients, mix well:

3/8 cup sesame tahini or raw
   nut butter
2 tsp. Chef Bonneau's
   Aminotone (optional) —
   obtainable at Health Food
   Stores

Then add 1-1/2 cups alfalfa sprouts. Serve over whole wheat toast, garnish with pimiento strips and ripe olives.

Salads

Of all the recommendations on diet in the Cayce readings one of the most invariable, it seems, is for raw fresh vegetables, as a salad, for the noon meal. Sometimes it was recommended that fruit salads be alternated with these (935-1). Frequently individuals were advised to prepare the raw vegetables often with gelatin (3429-1). Some were told not to use any acetic acid or synthetic vinegar with them, "but use that vinegar which would be made from apples, that is apple cider cinegar" (935-1).

Oil dressings, such as olive oil with paprika with the yolk of a hard boiled egg worked in, were recommended.

All the nutritionists we know agree on the value of an abundance of raw fresh vegetables, with deep-green leaves being especially rich in vitamins A, C, E, K, P, B2, folic acid, eight or more B vitamins, iron, copper, magnesium, calcium and other minerals.

Fresh salad greens are, or should be, the basis for most salads. There are a larger number of these than many people realize, and variety may be obtained by different combinations of these as well as of the other ingredients of the salad. Greens which may be used raw for salads include the following:

Kale	Beet Greens	Chicory
Spinach	Finocchi	Bibb Lettuce
Dandelion Greens	Chinese Cabbage	Savoy Cabbage
Field Salad	Iceburg Lettuce	Escarole
Water Cress	Mustard Greens	Celery
Boston Lettuce	Nasturtium Leaves	Romaine
Sour Grass	Green Cabbage	Leaf Lettuce
Turnip Greens	French Endive	

Eggplant Salad

1 medium-size eggplant	2 tbsp. salad oil
1 medium-size onion, grated	2 tbsp. minced parsley
Juice of one onion	

Bake eggplant, whole, in moderate oven (300°-350°) for 30-45 min. in glass dish. Cool and peel. Cut into cubes. Mix other ingredients and chill thoroughly before serving.

Jerusalem Artichoke Salad

2 cups scrubbed artichokes,   1 onion
  cubed   Parsley sprigs

Grind or chop finely and serve on bed of Romaine. Dressing may be added if desired.

Lettuce and Watercress Salad

2/3 cup nut meats   1/4 cup lemon juice
1 cup watercress   2 cups shredded lettuce

On a bed of watercress and shredded lettuce, serve nut meats (walnuts, pecans, almonds) which have been dipped in lemon juice.

Green and Gold Vegetable Bowl

1 lb. cut green beans, cooked, 2 tbsp. lemon juice
  drained   1 tsp. minced onion
1 cup sliced celery   1 tsp. dried parsley flakes
2 lbs. sliced carrots, cooked, 1 tsp. brown sugar
  drained   1/2 tsp. salt
1/4 cup salad oil   Lettuce

Toss beans with celery in small bowl, place carrots in a second bowl. Mix salad oil, lemon juice, onion, parsley flakes, sugar and salt in a cup, drizzle half over carrots and remaining half over beans; toss each lightly. Chill. Spoon carrot and bean mixture in separate piles in a lettuce-lined shallow serving bowl. Serve with mayonnaise or salad dressing as desired.

Riviera Green Beans

2 cups tender green beans cut in inch lengths
1 tbsp. green onions, chopped
1 young carrot, sliced thin on a grater
1 cup tiny red or yellow vine-ripened tomatoes
1/2 cup shelled peas
Salad greens and fresh herbs

All ingredients are raw. Line a salad bowl with the salad greens. Dice the fresh herbs over them. Toss the other ingredients together with your favorite dressing and pour them into the salad greens. Garnish with rose hips and paprika. Keep covered in refrigerator until serving time.

Raw Vegetable Salad

1 bunch spinach
2 green onions
1 vine-ripened tomato
4 sprigs watercress
1 small cucumber
1 carrot
Radishes to garnish

Chop spinach, onions, watercress, cucumber. Dice tomato and grate carrot. Combine all in mixing bowl and toss with mayonnaise. Make radish roses for garnish.

Cooked Vegetable Salad

1 cup carrots, cooked and cut in strips
1 cup string beans, cooked
1 cup lima beans, cooked
1 cup peas, cooked
Ripe olives for garnish

Cut the string beans through the center, lengthwise. Place all vegetables in 3/4 cup lemon honey dressing. Place combined vegetables in individual salad bowls and garnish with ripe olives.

Crisp Alfalfa Sprout Toss

2 cups finely cut celery
1 cup sprouted alfalfa

1 cup raisins
2 carrots, grated

Mix ingredients thoroughly and when ready to serve, make a "dent" in top of salad to fill with generous amounts of thick yogurt or sour cream.

Bean Sprout Tomato Salad

1 head Romaine lettuce
1 cucumber, sliced
3 tomatoes, vine-ripened

2 cups bean sprouts
Radishes
Ripe olives

Place Romaine leaves on salad plates. Place a layer of bean sprouts on the leaves. Slice alternate layers of cucumber and tomato over them, tapering up to a peak. Garnish with ripe olives and radishes. Serve with sour cream dressing.

Refreshing Alfalfa Sprout Slaw

3/4 cup crushed pineapple,
  unsweetened

3 cups cabbage, chopped
1 cup alfalfa sprouts

Mix ingredients and serve with remaining pineapple juice, unsweetened, as dressing.

Alfalfa Sprout Salad

2 cups alfalfa sprouts
3/4 cup avocado, cubed

1 cup sliced okra
3/4 cup green soy beans

Place lettuce leaves on salad plates. Mix above ingredients together and place mixture on the leaves. Top with slices of vine-ripened tomatoes. Serve with your favorite dressing.

Basic Recipe for Gelatin for Vegetable Salads

1 tbsp. gelatin
1/2 cup cold water
1 cup boiling water or light-
colored stock
1 tbsp. onion, grated

2 to 4 tbsp. honey
1/4 tsp. salt, if water is used
1/4 cup lemon juice
2 cups diced vegetables, cooked
or raw

Soak gelatin in cold water and dissolve thoroughly in boiling water or stock. Add honey, salt, lemon juice, and onion if desired. Chill. When about set, add vegetables, and chill until set firmly. Serve on lettuce leaves with mayonnaise.

Gelatin and Alfalfa Sprout Salad

4 tbsp. unflavored gelatin
1/2 cup warm water
1-1/2 cups pineapple juice
3/4 cup crushed pineapple,
unsweetened

1 cup alfalfa sprouts, chopped
3/4 cup diced avocado
2 tbsp. honey

Soften gelatin in warm water for five minutes. Liquefy with 1 cup unsweetened pinapple juice. Cook for few minutes, until gelatin is completely dissolved. Add remaining pineapple juice and honey. Let stand a few minutes, add chopped sprouts, avocado and pineapple. Pour into mold, chill, and serve topped with mayonnaise.

Alfalfa Sprout-Gelatin Salad

1 envelope unflavored gelatin
1/2 cup cold water
1 pint boiling water
1 lemon, juiced
1/2 cup honey

1 cup cabbage, finely shredded
1 cup celery, cut fine
1/4 cup green pepper,
chopped
1 cup alfalfa sprouts

Soak gelatin in cold water for five minutes. Add lemon juice, boiling water, honey and seasoning. Pour into mold. When beginning to set, add remaining ingredients. When firmly set, cut into squares and serve on lettuce leaves.

Alfalfa Sprout-Vegetable Gelatin Salad

1 envelope unflavored gelatin
1/2 cup cold water
1 pint boiling water
Juice of 1 lemon
1 cup carrots, shredded
1/2 cup green pepper, chopped
1/2 cup cucumber, thinly sliced
1/2 cup radishes, thinly sliced
1 cup alfalfa sprouts
1 teaspoon seasoning
1/2 cup honey

Soak gelatin in cold water for 5 minutes. Add lemon juice, boiling water, honey and seasoning. Pour into mold. When beginning to set, add remaining ingredients. Chill. Serve on lettuce.

Fresh Vegetable-Gelatin Salad

2 envelopes unflavored gelatin
1/2 cup cold water
2 cups hot water
1/3 cup honey
1-1/4 tsp. salt
1/4 cup lemon juice
2/3 cup ripe olives, pitted and diced
1-1/2 cups cabbage, shredded
3/4 cup celery, diced
3/4 cup carrots, shredded
1/4 cup green pepper, chopped
2 tbsp. pimiento, diced

Soften gelatin in cold water, add hot water and stir until dissolved. Stir in honey and next 2 ingredients; cool. Add olives and remaining ingredients; mix well. Pour into 1-1/4 qt. ring mold or 8x8x2 cake pan. Chill until firm. Cut into squares. Garnish with crisp greens and serve with mayonnaise. Serves 10-12.

Fresh Fruit Salad or Dessert

Use all your favorite fresh fruits (except pineapple and apples) with unflavored gelatin, for delicious flavor and Nature's own vitamin content.

1 envelope unflavored gelatin	1/2 cup grapefruit juice
1/4 cup cold water	1/8 tsp. salt
1 cup hot water	1 tbsp. lemon juice
1/4 cup honey	Fresh fruit, cut up

Soften gelatin in cold water, add honey, salt and hot water. Stir until dissolved. Add grapefruit and lemon juice. Mix well. Pour 1 cup mixture into mold that has been rinsed in cold water. When it begins to thicken, arrange fruit in it. Chill remaining gelatin until it begins to thicken, then whip until frothy and thick and pour on the gelatin mixture. Chill until firm. Serves 6.

Gelatin Fruit Salad

1 envelope unflavored gelatin	1 tbsp. coconut, finely grated
1-1/2 cups pineapple juice, unsweetened	2 tbsp. banana, cut fine
	2 tbsp. pineapple, unsweetened
1 tbsp. lemon juice	1 tbsp. orange, cut fine

Dissolve gelatin in 1/2 cup boiling water. Place on stove and let boil for 1 minute, stirring constantly. Add pineapple and lemon juice. Set aside to cool and when it is half set, add the mixed fruit and coconut. Pour into molds; it will set in approx. 20 min.

Tomato Aspic

4 pkgs. unflavored gelatin
2 cups cold tomato juice
5 cups hot tomato juice

1 tsp. salt
1/4 tsp. Tabasco
4 tbsp. lemon juice

Soften gelatin in cold tomato juice. Dissolve thoroughly in very hot tomato juice, stirring well. Season with salt, Tabasco and lemon juice. Pour into individual molds. When set, unmold on salad greens. Serve with salad dressing or plain. Serves 12.

Tomato-Shrimp Aspic

2 pkgs. gelatin, unflavored
1/2 cup cold water
2 cups tomato juice
3 tsp. lemon juice

Salt and pepper
1 cup celery, chopped
1/2 cup green olives, chopped
1/2 cup shrimp

Sprinkle gelatin on 1/2 cup water to soften. Place over very low heat and stir until dissolved. Remove from heat and stir in tomato juice and seasoning. Chill mixture to unbeaten egg-white consistency. Fold in celery, olives and shrimp. Turn into a 6-cup mold.

Shrimp Tossed Salad

1/4 cup salad oil
1-1/2 tbsp. lemon juice
1 tsp. salt
1/8 tsp. pepper
1/8 tsp. dry mustard
1/8 tsp. celery seeds
1/4 tsp. onion, grated

1/2 cup ripe olives, sliced
1 vine-ripened tomato, medium size, diced
1 cup cleaned, cooked fresh shrimp, crab meat or lobster
1 qt. crisp lettuce, coarsely shredded

Combine oil and next 6 ingredients. Mix well with fork. Place with remaining ingredients in salad bowl, pour dressing over all and toss. Serves 4-6.

Tuna Fish-Gelatin Salad

3 7-oz. cans tuna fish
4 hard boiled eggs, chopped
1 cup ripe olives, chopped
1 small onion, minced

1 cup celery, diced
2 pkgs. unflavored gelatin
1/2 cup cold water
3 cups mayonnaise

Combine first 5 ingredients. Soften gelatin in cold water and set over hot water and stir until dissolved. Stir in mayonnaise. Add to tuna mixture and blend well. Turn into mold. Chill until firm. Unmold and garnish with parsley and celery curls. Serves 12.

Crab-Stuffed Avocado

1/2 cup mayonnaise
1/2 cup celery, minced
1/4 cup pimiento, minced
2 tsp. lemon juice
1/8 tsp. Worcestershire
Dash Tabasco—(optional)

1-1/2 cups chilled cooked or
    canned crab or lobster meat
2 ripe avocados
Salt
Lemon juice

Combine first 6 ingredients. Halve avocados lengthwise and remove pits, peel. Sprinkle with lemon juice and salt. Arrange on bed of crisp greens and fill halves with crab meat. Top with dressing. Serves 4.

Salad Dressings

Salad dressings should all be homemade rather than the commercial variety. They are used to enhance the salad but should also contribute to health. There is some question as to the advisability of using vinegar, though the number of readings prohibiting this is too small to be really conclusive. (Ap-

76

ple cider vinegar is recommended.) We prefer lemon juice where acidity is desired. Oil used may be olive oil, frequently recommended in the readings, or vegetable oils. Adelle Davis ("Let's Cook It Right" and "Let's Get Well") recommends using a mixture of vegetable oils, peanut, soy and sunflower, as each is high in a different essential fatty acid.

Avocados, used either in salad dressings or otherwise in the salad, are a nutritionally valuable addition. They are rich in protein, in a highly digestible oil, and in vitamins A and C. Mineral contents include an ample amount of calcium, potassium, magnesium and sodium, considerable iron and phosphorus, and smaller amounts of manganese and copper, essential to the assimilation of iron.

Avocado Dressing

1 avocado   Juice of 1 orange or 1 lemon

Whip the avocado pulp to the consistency of whipped cream. Add citrus juice very gradually, then whip with a rotary beater until light and frothy.

Mayonnaise #1

Mayonnaise is a great favorite, not only as a dressing but for combining with other foods. Care must be used in storing all mayonnaise combinations in refrigerator, as they are subject to bacterial activity which may be very toxic without showing any evidence of spoilage.

Use chilled ingredients. Place in a medium-sized bowl and beat with a wire whisk: Beat in

2 egg yolks   1/4 to 1/2 tsp. dry mustard
1/2 tsp. salt   1/2 tsp. lemon juice
Few grains cayenne

Beat in very slowly, 1/2 tsp. at a time—1/2 cup salad oil —soy, safflower, peanut, etc. Place in a cup 3-1/2 tbsp. lemon juice.

Beat into dressing, 1/2 tsp. at a time—1/2 cup salad oil.

Alternate the oil with a few drops of lemon juice. If the ingredients are cold and are added slowly during constant beating this will make a good thick dressing. Should the dressing separate, place 1 egg yolk in a bowl, stir constantly and add the dressing very slowly. If the dressing is too heavy, thin it with cream or whipped cream.

When making mayonnaise with an electric beater, beat the egg yolks at medium speed for 4 min. Combine the dry ingredients and add them. Add 1-1/2 tbsp. cold water. Add 1/2 of the oil, drop by drop. When the dressing begins to thicken, add the lemon juice. Add the remaining oil more freely, beating constantly at medium speed. Time required, 20 min.

Mayonnaise #2

2 egg yolks	2 tbsp. lemon juice
1/2 tsp. salt	

Put above ingredients in electric blender or use electric mixer. Slowly add 3/4 cup oil while machine is running, until desired consistency. Add 2 tsp. honey for use on fruit salads.

Mayonnaise #3

2 egg yolks	1 tsp. honey
2 tbsp. lemon juice	Dash red pepper
1/2 tsp. salt	3/4 cup salad oil
1/2 tsp. dry mustard	

Blend all ingredients, except oil, in blender or mixer. Add salad oil very slowly, blending until thick.

French Dressing

1 cup salad oil	1 tsp. salt
1/3 cup lemon juice	1/4 tsp. garlic salt
1/4 tsp. pepper	

Put above ingredients into blender or mixer, and blend for 1 minute.

Almond Nut Dressing

2 tbsp. almond butter   4 tbsp. raw cream or milk

Beat together with an egg beater. This is an excellent dressing for fruits as well as vegetable salads.

Tomato Dressing

1 pt. canned tomatoes	2 tbsp. onion, grated
3/4 cup lemon juice	1 tsp. vegetable broth powder
1/2 cup salad oil	1 tsp. paprika
1/4 cup honey	2 cloves garlic
1 tbsp. soy sauce	

Sieve tomatoes and add next 7 ingredients. Place in quart jar, shake well, and add 2 whole cloves of garlic. This will keep indefinitely in your refrigerator. Yield: about 1 quart.

Peanut Butter Dressing

2 tbsp., cold pressed,
   unhydrogenated peanut
   butter

1 tbsp. salad oil
1-1/2 tbsp. lemon juice
1 cup mayonnaise

Mix all ingredients together.

Yogurt or Sour Cream Dressing

1 cup sour cream or yogurt   1/2 cup lemon juice

Mix together. This dressing is best with fruit salads, but may be used on vegetable salads also.

Yogurt and Honey Dressing

1 cup yogurt   Honey to taste

Mix and use as dressing on fruit salads.

Carob, Soy and Peanut Flours

Carob, soy and peanut flours are all alkaline-producing in the body. In most cases they would be used in combination with wheat flour which, being a starch, has an acid reaction. Cakes, cookies, etc. made with these are therefore not likely to be alkaline-producing, but would be less acid-producing than those made with the starchy flour alone.

Besides their alkaline-producing characteristics, these flours have much to recommend them, as their use provides another way of obtaining those properties recommended, or avoiding those warned against in the readings.

Carob flour is produced from the pod of the carob tree, or honey locust, and is thought by some to have been the "locust" that John the Baptist ate in the wilderness, thus called "St. John's Bread." It has a sweet taste and pleasant flavor, somewhat like chocolate, and may be used as substitute for both sugar and chocolate. It is low in starch and very high in natural sugars. It contains a large amount of minerals and a fair amount of several of the vitamins.

Soy flour is more than 33% protein, is extremely high in calcium, (200 mg. per cup), has more iron, thiamin, riboflavin and niacin than whole wheat flour, and is high in pantothenic acid, another important part of the Vitamin-B complex.

Peanut flour is higher yet in protein, one cup of flour (113 gm.) having 59 gm. of protein. It is also higher in calcium and thiamin than whole wheat flour, and has twice the amount of iron and riboflavin and more than 3 times the amount of niacin as does whole wheat. Peanut flour has the added advantage that it can be used raw, and has a flavor very pleasing to most people.

CHAPTER 5:   MEATS AND MEAT SUBSTITUTES

No reason seems to be given in the Cayce readings for the frequent recommendation of fish, fowl and lamb, rather than of red meats. However, since beef juice was often advised in cases of illness, it seems most likely that the reason is one of digestibility, rather than that of "vibrations" or such. It is recognized by nutritionists that fish, fowl and lamb are easily digested meats and that they are a good source of complete proteins. Fish, especially ocean varieties, also contain valuable minerals, particularly phosphorus and iodine, either not found in other meats, or occurring in smaller quantities.

The readings, likewise, give no reason for the statement that "any wild game is preferable even to other meats" (2514-4). J.I. Rodale, in "The Health Finder" states in support of his opinion that fish is an especially good food,—"First of all there has been no tampering with it. Commercial fertilizers and insecticides play no part in the fish business . . . Ocean fish cannot be doped, chemicalized or processed." The same things, of course, could be said of wild game, and may have resulted in that preference in the readings.

Glandular meats, as tripe, calf's liver, brains, and the like were referred to and recommended as "of the blood-building type" (275-25). Here we have the full agreement of the nutritionists. The vitamins found more abundantly in the glandular meats than in muscle are those needed to enable the bone marrow to produce red blood cells.

All meats should be cooked at low temperatures for maximum nutritive value, digestibility and flavor. High temperatures toughen the protein and cause contraction of the fibers, squeezing out the meat juices. Fish and glandular meats especially should be cooked at very low temperatures. These have very thin sheets of connective tissue which begin breaking down around 150°, and when they are cooked above

150° much of the juices will have been lost. Adding salt during cooking also results in juices being drawn out.

Meats should usually be roasted, baked, or broiled—never fried. Stewing is permissible if the broth is to be used, in which case a closely covered utensil should be used, and the meat should be simmered rather than boiled.

Temperatures and Time for Broiling

	Broiling Temp.	Thickness or cut	Time (Min.)
Fish steaks or fillets	Very Low	1 to 1-1/2 inches	15-18
Chicken, fryer or broiler	Low	Quartered or halved	45-50
Kidneys	Very Low	1/2 in.	12-16
Lamb chops, patties or steaks	Low	1 in.	20-30
	Low	2 in.	40-45
Milt	Low	Uncut	15-18
Rabbit, young fryer, 2 lbs.	Low	Quartered	45-50
Liver	Low	3/4 in.	12-18
Brains	Low	3/4 in.	15-20

Temperatures and Time for Baking or Roasting

	Oven Temp.	Internal Temp. at which served	Time (Min. per lb.)
Whole fish or fillets	300°	140°	1 in. thick-20 2 in. thick-30 3 in. thick-35
Chicken, roasting	300°	185°	35-40
Chicken, stewing	225°	185°	60-70
Duck, young	300°	185°	25-30
Goose, young	300°	185°	25-30
Lamb, leg	300°	155°-160°	25-30
Lamb, shoulder	275°	155°-160°	40-45
Rabbit	300°	180°	30-35
Turkey, large	300°	180°-185°	15-18
Turkey, small	300°	180°-185°	20-25
Liver, uncut	300°	145°-160°	15-20

Curried Cod Bake

2 lbs. frozen cod, partly thawed
2 large onions, chopped
  (2 cups)
1 clove garlic, minced
2 tbsp. butter
3 med. size apples, pared,
cored, quartered and sliced
6 oz. tomato paste
3/4 cup water
2 tsp. salt
1 tsp. curry powder
1/8 tsp. pepper

Cut cod into 6 serving pieces, place in a 6-cup shallow baking dish. Sauté onions and garlic in butter or margarine until soft in a medium-size frying pan; stir in remaining ingredients. Heat, stirring constantly, to boiling; spoon over fish and cover. Bake in moderate oven (350°) 1-1/2 hour, or until fish flakes easily.

Poached Eggs and Broiled Fish

For a treat, the eggs may be poached in muffin tins which have been well oiled so that the eggs come out easily. Arrange the muffin-shaped eggs on a platter and surround them with chunks of broiled fish. This is a rare protein treat, as broiled fish is one of the highest sources of protein obtainable, and eggs are a fine source of minerals and vitamins as well as protein. Garnish with paprika.

Salmon Loaf

1 can salmon
1 tsp. lemon juice
1 can celery soup
3 tsp. parsley, chopped
3 tsp. green pepper, chopped
1 cup cooked peas
Dash nutmeg

Bake in moderate oven (350°) for 30 min.

Quick-Baked Frozen Fish Fillets

This exception to the rule that fish is better when fresh, or thawed before cooking, is inserted for the benefit of the hurry-up cook.

Cut into quarters 1 lb.—block frozen fillets.
Combine 1/4 cup unbleached flour
　　　　　3/4 tsp. salt
　　　　　1/8 tsp. pepper

Roll the fish in this until well coated, then place in a well-greased oven-proof dish.

Sauté lightly 1 tsp. grated onion in 3 tbsp. melted butter and add 1/2 cup vegetable stock.

Pour the sauce over the fish, cover closely and bake in 300° oven for 20 to 25 min.

Red Snapper Fish Fillets

1-1/4 lb. red snapper fillets
2 cans tomato sauce, Spanish style
1 tbsp. onion, minced
1 tbsp. parsley, minced
Dash Cayenne

Place the fish fillets in oiled baking dish. Pour tomato sauce over them. Sprinkle with onion, parsley and cayenne. Place in preheated 300° oven for about 25 min. or until fillets are done. Serves 5.

Fillet of Sole with Tomato-Herb Dressing

Rub a warm skillet lightly with butter. Then slowly sauté 3 tbsp. finely minced onion and 1 tbsp. finely chopped green pepper until tender. Stir in:

Juice of 1 lime	1/2 tsp. oregano
2 tbsp. tomato paste	Pinch of savory
1 can homemade mayonnaise	

Place 4 sole fillets on a broiler pan, sprinkle with lime juice, salt and cracked pepper and broil until just heated through (about 5 min.). Serve topped with some of the sauce and the remainder in separate bowl. Makes 4 servings.

Baked Fish with Sour Cream

Split and remove bones from—
  4 lb. whitefish

Flatten it out and rub inside and out with
  paprika and butter

Place it on an oven-proof dish or shallow baking pan under a flame until it is lightly browned. Cover with
  2 cups sour cream

Place a lid over it and bake in 300° oven for 25 to 35 min. Remove from oven and season with salt.

Celery-Broiled Chicken

Rub 2 young broilers, split lengthwise, all over with lemon juice, then sprinkle with cracked pepper. Place skin side down on a broiler pan, lay strips of celery in the cavities and broil for 10 to 12 min. Turn skin side up, lay fresh celery strips over all and broil until browned and tender. Makes 4 servings.

Broiled Chicken Fryers

Have the chicken cut in serving pieces. Rub the outside with a mixture of salt and poultry seasoning and place the pieces on the broiler rack. Broil low in the oven until browned, turn and finish broiling.

Stewed Chicken

Select a young chicken which has a small amount of fat, and stew it with a big handful of celery tops, plus salt. Use a small amount of water, cook it gently, letting the water nearly cook away. Serve hot. It is a most delightful meat when prepared this way.

Chinese Turkey

15 lb. turkey	1 cup honey
Soy sauce	3/4 cup butter, unsalted

Dress the turkey, wiping the interior with soy sauce, and stuff with dressing, (below). Preheat oven to 450°. Make a paste of honey and butter and completely plaster the bird with this mixture, being careful to get it in under the wings. Place the turkey in a large pan and into the hot oven for 1/2 hr. until it is evenly colored. Turn it several times with wooden spoons, being careful not to break the skin. Continue to brown until it is evenly crusted to a blackish brown. The honey turns black and in carbonizing completely seals the skin. Reduce the heat to 300° and roast for 3 to 4 hours. Baste with drippings after the first hour of cooking and every 20 min. afterward.

Dressing

16 ribs celery, leaves and stem cut up	1 cup onion, lightly sautéed
1 cup parsley, chopped	1 cup mushrooms, lightly sautéed
24 Julienne strips tangerine rind	

Roast Duck

3-1/2 to 4 lb. domestic duck	1/2 tsp. salt
1 orange, unsprayed	1 tsp. honey
1/2 cup boiling consommé	1 tsp. lemon juice
3 tsp. brown sugar	Currant jelly

Prepare the duck for cooking. Place it unstuffed on a rack in a pan in a moderate oven (325°). Roast the duck uncovered, allowing 20 to 30 min. to the pound. Skin the orange and scrape the white pulp from the skin with a spoon and discard it. Cut the yellow peel into very thin strips. Add a cupful of boiling water and simmer the peel for 15 min. Drain it. Reserve the liquid. Remove all membrane from the orange sections and discard it. Fifteen minutes before the duck is done, pour the drippings from the pan and replace with the consommé. Continue to cook the duck and add to the drippings the orange liquid, salt, honey and lemon juice. Simmer these ingredients for 10 min. Add the currant jelly and stir until dissolved. Add the orange peel and simmer 10 min. longer. Add the consommé from the pan. Sprinkle the orange sections with the brown sugar and broil them for 3 min. Cut the duck into individual servings. Arrange on a hot platter and garnish with orange sections and dabs of currant jelly. Pour the sauce over it.

Roast Goose with Apple Dressing

Prepare on 8 lb. goose for cooking. (This weight is for a bird dressed but not drawn). Rub the inside with salt and fill with following dressing:

Peel, quarter and core cooking applies and combine them with currants or raisins, about 1 cup to 6 cups apples. Steam the currants or raisins in 2 tbsp. water in top of double boiler for 15 min. before combining.

Allow a cupful of dressing to each pound of bird. If the bird is very fat, prick through the skin into the fat layer around the legs and wings. Truss the goose. Roast in moderate oven (325°) allowing 25 min. to the pound, on a rack in an uncovered pan.

Chicken Cantonese

2 frying chickens, disjointed
1/4 cup honey
1/4 cup soy sauce

1/2 cup catsup
1/4 cup lemon juice

Arrange chicken pieces in single layer in large baking dish. Mix honey, soy sauce, catsup and lemon juice. Pour over chicken pieces. Allow chicken to stand in marinade several hours or over night. Cover pan and bake in 325° oven 1 hr. Remove cover and baste with sauce. Return to oven and bake uncovered until tender.

Roast Leg of Lamb

Place the leg of lamb on a roaster rack with the fat side up. Rub it heavily with sea kelp. If you like mint with lamb, then cut through the fat at intervals and pack mint leaves in the cuts. If you prefer other herbs, use them instead of the mint. Bake in a 300° oven, allowing 25 to 30 min. per lb.

Broiled Lamb Chops and Potatoes

Prepare the chops in the morning and keep refrigerated in a covered dish. If you leave any fat on, cut every 1/2 in. to prevent curling. Brush each chop with cooking oil, then sprinkle with either dried mint leaves or dried herbs and sea kelp. A suitable herb is marjoram. Stack the chops so that they are seasoned from both top and bottom through the day. Later, place them on the broiler rack at room temperature while you prepare the potatoes. Scrub, but do not peel the potatoes and cut in thin slices. Arrange them on the broiler rack around the lamb chops; then brush with cooking oil and sprinkle with sea kelp. Broil the chops and potatoes slowly, turning the chops when browned on one side. Just before turning off the broiler, sprinkle the potato slices with sesame seeds and let them toast slightly. Serve chops and potatoes very hot.

Liver Dumplings and Dill Sauce

Put 2 cups of liver through a food grinder. Add the following ingredients:

2 heaping tbsp. corn meal	1 tsp. fresh or dried marjoram
2 eggs, beaten	2 tsp. sea kelp
1 tsp. minced onion	

This will make a stiff dumpling dough. In a large kettle, put 3 cups of meat and vegetable stock and place over medium heat. When it boils, dip a large tablespoon into the broth, then dip up a heaping spoonful of the dumpling batter, shaping it into a round ball with the spoon. Drop it into the boiling broth; dip the spoon in the broth again and repeat until you have 8 or 9 round liver dumplings distributed evenly in the boiling broth. Cover tightly and cook gently for 15 min. without lifting the cover.

Lift the dumplings out with a slotted spoon and place them in a rather deep serving dish. Keep warm. Put 2 tbsp. of fat green dill seed (from the freezer if they aren't available in the garden as yet) in the broth. Thicken it with 2 rounded tbsp. of arrowroot flour moistened in cold water. Pour this dill gravy over the liver dumplings and serve very hot.

This is an excellent way to serve liver. The dumplings are very tender and can be eaten by small children and elderly people.

Braised Liver

2 lb. liver (1 thick piece)	2 tbsp. catsup
2 tsp. cooking oil	1 tbsp. green pepper, chopped
1 onion, sliced	Salt and pepper
2 tsp. Worcestershire sauce	Hot water

Place liver in greased baking dish and brush sides with oil. Add remaining ingredients, using enough hot water to nearly cover liver. Place lid on and cook at 300° for about 1-1/2 hrs. Remove lid for last 15 min. Serves 6.

Chicken-Livers Mold

Boil chicken livers in water to which a handful of celery leaves and sea kelp has been added. Strain the broth and keep it for use as liquid for a molded or pressed meat dish later. Chop livers fine and add your own mayonnaise. Place in a mold and chill. Serve with a sprinkling of chopped egg and onion rings.

Baked Brains

1 pair lamb or beef brains	1 tbsp. lemon juice
3 tbsp. water	

Place all ingredients in saucepan and simmer for 15 min., to prepare brains for recipe.

1 pair prepared brains, chopped coarsely	4 tbsp. cream
	1 tbsp. catsup
1/4 cup bread crumbs, whole wheat	1/2 tbsp. lemon juice
	1/3 tsp. salt
2 hard-cooked eggs, chopped	1/8 tsp. pepper or paprika

Place all ingredients in a greased baking dish or in individual dishes. Sprinkle the top with additional whole wheat bread crumbs. Dot generously with butter. Bake for 15 min. at 400°.

Broiled Calf Brains on Tomatoes

Prepare brains according to directions in preceding recipe.

2 sets of calf brains, spread with butter	Seasoning of salt, pepper, brown sugar and whole wheat bread crumbs
8 thick slices of vine-ripened tomatoes	

Place prepared butter-spread brains on the greased rack of broiler pan. Broil them for 5 min. on one side. Place tomato slices on an oven-proof plate; season tomato slices with salt, pepper and brown sugar and cover one side with buttered whole wheat bread crumbs. Place the brains, cooked side down, on the tomatoes. Broil them for 5 min. longer, and serve at once.

Wild Game, Rabbit, Pheasant

Cut rabbit into serving pieces, after tendons of left legs have been removed; season with salt, flour and brown quickly in oil. Arrange pieces in roaster pan and spread with sauce made with the following:

1/2 cup sour cream	1/2 cup water
Juice of 1 lemon	

Bake uncovered at 300° allowing 35 to 45 min. per lb. In the meantime, sauté 1/2 lb. mushrooms in 1/4 cup butter for about 5 min. Remove rabbit from pan and arrange on large platter. Add about 1 cup water to pan and heat in order to get all the juices from the meat. In a bowl mix 1 cup sour cream, 1/2 cup water and 2 tbsp. whole wheat flour and add this to the meat juices to make a light gravy. Add mushrooms to the gravy and season to taste.

Complete proteins, that is, those containing all the essential amino acids, are necessary for building body tissue and thus maintaining health. Also, many of the vitamins necessary to health can be produced in the body itself only if a sufficient supply of these amino acids is obtained. It is rather difficult to obtain a sufficient amount of complete proteins without including meat or at least eggs and dairy products in the diet. The following table gives the approximate amounts of complete proteins from animal and vegetable sources:

Animal —	Amount	Gms. Protein
Milk, whole, skim, buttermilk	1 qt.	32 to 35
Cottage cheese	½ cup	20
American or Swiss cheese	1 oz.	7
Meat, fish or fowl, boned	¼ lb.	18 to 22
Egg	1	6
Vegetable —	Amount	Gms. Protein
Soybean flour	1 cup	60
Cottonseed flour	1 cup	60
Wheat germ	1 cup	48
Brewer's yeast, powdered	¼ cup	25
Soy beans, cooked	½ cup	20
Nuts	½ cup	14 to 22

The protein of some nuts is incomplete; others are either complete or on the borderline. Peanuts, for example, can support growth and maintenance, aaccording to Adelle Davis[1], but not reproduction.

It is possible to obtain all the essential amino acids from incomplete proteins by combining foods which together have all the essentials. If these are taken at the same meal they may be used by the body as complete proteins. Baked beans and brown bread, for instance, together supply all the essential amino acids, but the amount of protein supplied by the quantity of these normally eaten would not be very large. Also, considerable study would be required concerning the composition of the various protein foods,—that is, which amino acids each contained,—in order to have any degree of certainty as to the amount of complete protein obtained in this way.

[1] "Let's Eat Right To Keep Fit"

Therefore it is very important that as much as possible of the complete protein foods be included in any meatless diet.

Meat Substitutes

Carrot Loaf

1 cup mashed cooked carrots	2 cups cooked rice
1 small grated onion	1/2 can tomato paste
2 tbsp. oil or butter	2 eggs
1/2 cup peanut butter	

Combine all above ingredients as you would for a meat loaf. Do not overcook the rice. Reserve the other portion of the tomato paste to make the sauce to serve with the loaf. Bake at 350° for 1 hr.

Sauce

2 tbsp. butter	Dash pepper
2 tbsp. flour (or cornstarch)	1 cup cold water
1/2 tsp. salt	1/2 can tomato paste

You can also add 2 tbsp. chopped parsley if you have it, or just garnish it with parsley for color.

Carrot Burgers

1 cup raw carrot, grated	1 tbsp. fresh herbs, coarsely chopped
1 cup walnuts, ground, or your local variety	2 egg yolks, raw
1 cup sunflower seeds, ground	Raw peanut flour

Blend all ingredients together, shape into patties and roll in raw peanut flour. Keep in tightly covered dish until served.

Asparagus Soufflé

1 pt. canned asparagus or equal
  amount fresh cooked
3 egg yolks

Salt
1 cup cream
2 tbsp. butter

Put asparagus through collander. Blend pulp and liquid with well-beaten egg yolks and cream. Salt to taste and place in individual oiled molds. Place molds in pan to which 1/4 in. water has been added and bake in moderate oven until custard is set. Add butter to each mold. Serve hot.

Sweet Potato Souffle

2 cups sweet potato, baked
2 eggs, separated

1 tsp. salt
2/3 cup cream

Mash baked sweet potato and blend with beaten egg yolks, salt and cream. Fold in stiffly beaten egg whites and bake 30 min. in moderate oven.

Vegetable Loaf

2 lbs. raw spinach
1-1/2 cups raw carrots, grated
1 onion, chopped
1 cup celery, diced

1 green pepper, chopped
1/2 cup nut meats
2 eggs, beaten
1/2 cup vegetable oil

Mix vegetables and steam together, then add 1/2 cup nut meats, chopped well. Mix beaten eggs and oil and add to mixture. Bake in moderate oven approximately 1/2 hr. Serve with tomato juice.

Walnut Lentil Loaf

1 cup lentils	1 tsp. vegetized salt
1 cup walnuts, chopped	1 egg
1/2 cup celery, chopped	1/2 cup milk
1 small onion, cut fine	

Combine lentils, walnuts, celery, onion and salt. Over these pour milk to which has been added beaten egg. Mix lightly. Bake in oiled casserole in moderate oven for 1 hr.

Almond Nut Loaf

1 cup celery tops	1 cup apples
1 cup celery	1 egg
1 cup almonds	1/2 cup milk

Chop finely and blend the first four ingredients. Beat egg and add milk and mix lightly with other ingredients. Bake in oiled loaf pan in moderate oven for 1 hr.

Nut Loaf Surprise

1 onion, chopped	1 tsp. soy sauce
1 cup nut meats, chopped	Cottage cheese for desired
1/4 tsp. paprika	consistency
1-1/2 tsp. lemon juice	

Combine ingredients and form into loaf. Pack firmly and chill. Cut into slices and serve.

Nut Patties

2 cups cooked grated carrots	1/4 cup pecan butter (or
2 tbsp. minced parsley	other nut butter) thinned
1 tsp. vegetable broth powder	with water

Thin nut butter with water to the consistency of a very thick

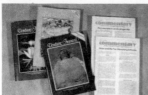

Discover the wealth of information in the Edgar Cayce readings

	ESP	Astrology
	Dreams	Atlantis
	Soul Mates	Psychic
Earth Changes	Karma	Numerology
Universal Laws	Reincarnation	Mysticism
Meditation	Akashic Records	Spiritual Healing
Holistic Health	Death and Dying	And other topics

Membership Benefits You Receive Each Month

- Magazine
- Home-study lessons
- Names of doctors and health care professionals in your area
- Library-by-mail
- Summer seminars
- Programs in your area
- Research projects
- Edgar Cayce medical readings on loan
- Notice of new Cayce-related books on all topics

Fill in and Mail This Card Today:

Yes, I want to know more about Edgar Cayce's *Association for Research & Enlightenment, Inc.* (A.R.E.®) (Check either or both boxes below.)

☐ Please send me more information.   `brc`

and/or

☐ Please send me a trial offer for membership.   `N31/PMZ`

Trial offer includes: magazine, free book, free research report, member packet. If at the end of 3 months' trial you wish to continue your membership, you need only pay the introductory membership level.

_____
Name (please print)

_____
Address

_____
City   State   Zip

 Or Call Today 1-800-368-2727

You may cancel at any time and receive a full refund on all unmailed benefits.

**EDGAR CAYCE FOUNDATION and
A.R.E. LIBRARY/CONFERENCE CENTER**
Virginia Beach, Va.
OVER 50 YEARS OF SERVICE

BUSINESS REPLY CARD
First Class Permit No. 2456, Virginia Beach, Va.

POSTAGE WILL BE PAID BY

A.R.E.®
P.O. Box 595
Virginia Beach, VA 23451

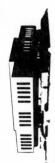

785-71

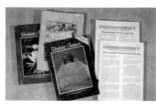

Discover the wealth of information in the Edgar Cayce readings

	ESP	Astrology
	Dreams	Atlantis
	Soul Mates	Psychic
Earth Changes	Karma	Numerology
Universal Laws	Reincarnation	Mysticism
Meditation	Akashic Records	Spiritual Healing
Holistic Health	Death and Dying	And other topics

Membership Benefits You Receive Each Month

- Magazine
- Home-study lessons
- Names of doctors and health care professionals in your area

- Library-by-mail
- Summer seminars
- Programs in your area
- Research projects

- Edgar Cayce medical readings on loan
- Notice of new Cayce-related books on all topics

Fill in and Mail This Card Today:

Yes, I want to know more about Edgar Cayce's *Association for Research & Enlightenment, Inc.* (A.R.E.®) (Check either or both boxes below.)

☐ Please send me more information.   `brc`
        and/or
☐ Please send me a trial offer for membership.   `N31/PMZ`

Trial offer includes: magazine, free book, free research report, member packet. If at the end of 3 months' trial you wish to continue your membership, you need only pay the introductory membership level.

_____

Name (please print)

_____

Address

_____
City   State   Zip

 Or Call Today 1-800-368-2727

You may cancel at any time and receive a full refund on all unmailed benefits.

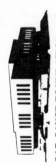

sauce. Mix well with other ingredients and shape into patties. Roll in whole wheat toast crumbs, place on buttered tin and bake in moderate oven until brown.

Nut Loaf

1 cup walnut meats, chopped fine	1 onion, chopped fine
1 cup whole wheat bread crumbs, dried	1 egg
	1/2 cup celery, chopped fine
1/2 cup wheat germ	1 clove garlic
	1/2 cup milk

Beat egg and add to milk. Pour this over the other ingredients and mix well. Bake in oiled loaf pan 1-1/2 hrs. in moderate oven.

Large Nut Roast

2 eggs	1 cup wheat germ
1 cup milk	1/2 cup celery, chopped
1/2 cup onion, minced	4 tbsp. butter
2 cups walnuts or pecans ground	1/2 tsp. powdered sage
	1 tbsp. parsley, chopped
1 cup whole wheat bread crumbs	Salt and dash of garlic

Pour 1/2 cup water in skillet and cook onion for 5 min. Beat eggs well, adding milk, then add to onion and remaining ingredients. Mix well and put in oiled baking dish. Cook 1/2 to 3/4 hr., basting with equal parts hot water and melted butter.

Spinach Nut Loaf

3 bunches cleaned spinach, cut
up
1 cup nut meats, chopped
2 eggs, well beaten
1 tsp. salt
1 small onion, diced finely

1 bunch parsley, small,
chopped finely
1/2 cup wheat germ
3/4 cup whole wheat bread
crumbs

Mix all but 1/2 cup bread crumbs. Place in oiled loaf pan.
Sprinkle remaining bread crumbs over top, dot with butter
and bake in moderate oven about 30 min. Serve with tomato
juice sauce.

Lima Bean Loaf

2 cups cooked lima beans
(fresh or dried)
1 cup whole wheat bread
crumbs
2 tbsp. melted butter, or oil
1/2 cup green peppers,
chopped

1/2 cup onions, chopped
1/2 cup nuts, chopped
2 eggs, well beaten
1/2 cup milk or cream
Vegetable salt to taste

Mix all ingredients together thoroughly, place in well-buttered
loaf pan and bake in a moderate oven for about 30 min. or
until done. Baste with melted butter.

Soybean Loaf #1

3 cups cooked soybeans,
seasoned
1/2 tsp. dry mustard

2 tsp. sorghum
2 tsp. raw sugar
1/2 cup hot water

Mash cooked soybeans and mold into loaf pan. Pour mixture
of remaining ingredients over loaf. Bake uncovered in
moderate oven until browned.

Soybean Noodles with Cheese

3 cups cooked soy noodles
2 tbsp. vegetable broth powder
1/2 cup cooked tomatoes

1/3 cup American cheese,
grated

Place noodles in oiled baking dish and pour tomatoes over them. Sprinkle broth powder over noodles and then cheese. Bake in moderate oven for 35 min.

Soybean Egg Loaf

1/2 lb. soybeans, cooked
2 eggs
2 tbsp. parsley, chopped

1/2 cup thinly sliced celery
1 small onion
2 tsp. salt

Put soybeans through grinder. Beat eggs well. Mix all ingredients and mold into loaf pan. Bake in moderate oven for 30 min.

Soybean Loaf #2

3 cups soybeans, cooked
1 small onion, chopped
1 tbsp. salad oil

1/2 cup cooked tomatoes
1/2 cup green pepper,
chopped

Mash cooked soybeans and mix with remaining ingredients. Season to taste and bake in oiled loaf pan for 1 hr. in moderate oven. Serve with tomato sauce.

Eggs in a Nest

1 egg
1/3 cup milk
4 slices whole wheat bread,
  slightly dry

2 tbsp. butter or margarine
1 pkg. (10 oz.) frozen spinach,
  cooked, drained and seasoned
4 eggs, poached

Beat egg slightly with milk in a pie plate. Dip bread slices in mixture, turning to soak both sides well. Sauté slowly in butter in a large frying pan until golden, turning once. Top each slice with a ring of spinach, place poached egg in center. Serve hot.

Cottage Cheese Patties

1 small onion, finely chopped
1 lb. cottage cheese
3/4 cup whole wheat bread
  crumbs

1/3 cup wheat germ

Mix ingredients and form into small patties and bake on greased baking sheet in moderate oven 20 min.

Cheese Loaf

2 tbsp. onion, chopped
2 tbsp. butter
1 cup walnuts or pecans,
  chopped
1/2 cup whole wheat bread
  crumbs

1/2 cup wheat germ
1 cup cheese, grated
2/3 cup hot water
2 tbsp. lemon juice
2 beaten eggs
Salt to taste

Cook onions in a little water for 5 min. Add all ingredients, then mix well. Put in well-oiled loaf pan and bake for 30 min. Serve with tomato juice sauce, if desired.

CHAPTER 6: WHOLE GRAIN BREADS
AND CEREALS

Wheat is, at least in the United States, the most popular grain for bread making, largely because its protein has the proper texture for forming gas bubbles, thereby making a light loaf. However, there are also nutritional advantages, provided whole wheat grain is used, including both the bran and germ. Wheat, unlike other grains, such as rye, will not grow on soil low in phosphorus, so all wheat has a fairly high content of this bone-building mineral, as well as silicon and iron. It is also an excellent source of the vitamin B complex, and wheat germ is the richest known source of vitamin E, so important in maintaining a healthy cardio-vascular system. There is considerable evidence of other factors in wheat, as yet unnamed, which play important parts in health and vitality.

Many diet outlines in the readings included whole grain cereals and bread. "Rolled or cracked whole wheat," one recommended, "not cooked too long so as to destroy the whole vitamin force—this will add to the body the proper portions of iron, silicon, and the vitamins necessary to build up the blood supply that makes for resistance in the system (840-1). Buckwheat cakes, rice cakes and graham (whole wheat) cakes were also frequently recommended.

It is of importance that whole wheat flour be freshly ground in order to protect the vitamin content. Deterioration of vitamins begins almost immediately after grinding, due to oxidation, and it is estimated that at least half the vitamin content may be lost within a few days' time, especially if the flour is not refrigerated. The oil of the wheat germ also becomes rancid in a short time, impairing the flavor. Cracked wheat used for cereal should also, of course, be cracked as shortly before use as possible. We recommend the purchase of a small hand mill for this purpose.

Bread Making

There are only two important secrets to making good whole wheat bread. The first is the type of flour used. Hard wheat should be used, and there is no substitute for fresh stone-ground flour for flavor, texture and nutritional value of the finished product.* Flour ground by roller mills contains larger particles of bran, which may be irritating to the digestive tract, makes bread of coarser texture, and the difference in flavor of freshly ground flour, as compared to that left standing for some time in warehouses and grocers' shelves, can hardly be imagined.

The second important secret is in allowing sufficient time after mixing and before baking for the bran particles to absorb the moisture and become soft. This requires at least four hours, preferably longer, and is necessary to prevent the bread from being crumbly and dry.

Other points are of lesser importance. The exact amount of flour needed to make dough of proper consistency for handling may vary if measured by volume, as it may be packed more in some cases than others (measurements in bread recipes are for unsifted flour) and the best degree of stiffness must be learned from experience. Weighing the flour, if possible, may give more uniform results.

The exact temperature at which bread rises (80° to 85°), is important only if you wish rising time to be as short as possible. If you have plenty of time, room temperature is usually quite satisfactory, and you avoid the danger of accidentally killing the yeast, which is possible from setting dough in too warm a place, as in an oven.

The exact amount of kneading can only be learned by experience. (It may vary with different flours). Time is important for the *best* possible texture in bread, but not essential for *good* bread. In short, it is difficult if good ingredients are used with a reasonable amount of care, not to have bread superior in flavor and nutrition, so don't hesitate to try because of lack of experience.

* If this kind of flour is not available, a small family size stone grinding mill would be a worthwhile investment. For information write to : Lee Engineering Company, 2023 W. Wisconsin Avenue, Milwaukee, Wisconsin, 53201

Whole Wheat Bread

5-1/3 cups lukewarm water
1 pkg. or cake yeast
2 tbsp. salt
1/3 cup vegetable oil

1/2 cup honey
3-1/2 lbs. (12 cups) unsifted
    whole wheat flour

Dissolve yeast in water, add salt, oil and honey, and stir. Add flour all at once and stir until thoroughly mixed, then let stand for 20 min. or longer before kneading. Knead on floured board until smooth and elastic and place in well-oiled bowl or pan (at least 6-qt. size). Cover (plastic wrap or a thin sheet of plastic is good for this) and let rise to double its bulk. Punch down well to remove all gas bubbles. Continue to let rise, punching down each time as soon as double in bulk until ready to make into loaves, preferably about 5 hrs. from time of mixing. It should rise at least twice in this time. Turn out on floured board, knead a few minutes and divide into 4 equal portions. Knead and form into loaves, place in well-greased medium size loaf pans, lightly grease top surface with vegetable oil, and cover loosely with plastic wrap. Let rise until not quite double in bulk and bake at 325° about 45 min.

Variations

#1 Dough may be mixed in the evening, using cold rather than lukewarm water and doubling the amount of yeast. Leave in the refrigerator over night. In morning remove from refrigerator and let stand at room temperature one-half hr., then knead and shape into loaves. Let rise and bake as in basic recipe.

#2 Mix in evening, omitting yeast, and let stand at room temperature over night. In morning, soften two yeast cakes or two packages dry yeast in 2 to 4 tbsp. warm water and add to dough mixture, working it in well with hands. Let dough rest 10 to 20 min. then knead, allowing to rise until double in bulk and then shape into loaves as above.

#3 If time does not allow for any of above methods, yeast may be increased to 2 or 3 cakes, dough left in warm place to rise (be sure temperature is not above 85°) and kneaded and shaped into loaves after rising once to double in bulk, about 45 min. or less. Bread will be less moist than in other methods.

#4 When bread has been formed into loaves, brush with water rather than oil and sprinkle with sesame seed. This adds a delightful flavor as well as added nutrition.

#5 For increasing nutritive value, milk may be substituted for water (if fresh milk is used it must be scalded), soy flour substituted for part of the whole wheat flour (not more than one-fourth the quantity, or 2 to 4 tbsp.) Brewer's yeast may be added, but bread will probably not be as light, as the addition of substances not containing gluten decreases the elasticity. Blackstrap molasses, which is extremely high in calcium, iron, and some of the B vitamins, may be substituted for all or part of the honey.

Whole Wheat Buns and Rolls

Buns and rolls may be made from the dough for whole wheat bread.

Hamburger Buns: Take pieces of dough the size of an egg. Roll into a ball and flatten to 3/4 in. thickness. Place on oiled cookie sheet or shallow pan, allowing at least 1 in. between buns; brush with vegetable oil, cover with plastic wrap and allow to rise until double or triple in size. Bake in moderate oven about 20 min.

Rolls: roll out on floured board to 1/2 in. thickness. Cut with biscuit cutter, dip in vegetable oil and place close together in baking pan. Cover, let rise and bake as above.

Parker House Rolls are shaped by holding left fore-finger across center of round, bringing far side of dough over and pressing edges together.

Refrigerator Rolls

1-1/2 cups lukewarm water	1/3 cup vegetable oil
2 pkgs. or cakes yeast	2 eggs, well beaten
2 tsp. salt	4-1/2 to 5 cups unsifted whole
1/3 cup honey	wheat flour

Dissolve yeast, salt and honey in lukewarm water. Add oil and eggs and mix well, then stir in flour. Set in refrigerator over night. Take dough from refrigerator about 2 hrs. before time for serving rolls, let stand at room temperature about 1/2 hr. Knead on floured board, shape, and let rise as above. Bake 15 to 20 min. at 375°.

Scalded fresh milk or reconstituted powdered skim milk may be substituted for 1 cup of the water in this recipe, in which case the yeast and honey should be dissolved in the water (1/2 cup) and allowed to stand 20 min. before adding other ingredients.

Wheat Germ Rolls

1 cup warm water or milk	1/4 cup vegetable oil
1 cake or pkg. yeast	3/4 cup toasted wheat germ
1-1/2 tsp. salt	1/3 cup powdered milk
3 tbsp. blackstrap molasses	2-1/2 cups whole wheat flour
1 egg	

Dissolve yeast in liquid, add other ingredients and stir to mix, then beat 200 strokes by hand or 10 min. with electric mixer. Cover bowl, set in warm place (not over 85°) until double in bulk. Make into rolls, kneading thoroughly and shaping as desired. When double or triple in bulk, bake at 350° for 20 to 25 min. or until brown.

If time allows, this dough may be placed in refrigerator over night as in recipe for Refrigerator Rolls, or after rising may be stirred down and left in refrigerator for 1 to 8 hrs. before using.

Potato Rolls

1-1/2 cups milk	2 eggs, beaten
1/2 cup potato water	1/3 cup mashed potato
2 pkgs. or cakes yeast	4 tbsp. vegetable oil
4 tbsp. honey	6 to 7 cups sifted whole wheat
2 tsp. salt	flour

Dissolve yeast in liquids, add honey, salt, eggs, oil and mashed potatoes. Mix well, and stir in 2-1/2 cups flour to make a sponge. Let rise 1/2 hr. Add about 3-1/2 cups flour to make a medium stiff dough. Knead well and let rise until double in bulk. Knead again and shape into rolls. Put on well-greased pans, let rise 1 to 1-1/2 hrs. and bake for 20 min. at 400°.

Cinnamon Rolls

Make dough as in either of foregoing recipes. Roll 1/4 in. thick, brush with mixture of melted butter and vegetable oil and dribble honey over surface. Sprinkle with cinnamon, and with raisins or pecans or walnuts if desired. Roll like jelly roll, cut in 1-in. pieces and set close together in baking pan. Let rise and bake in moderate oven.

Coffee Cake

Add 1/4 cup raw sugar or extra honey and 1/2 cup raisins to roll dough. After dough rises roll it 1/3 in. thick, brush surface with molasses or honey, sprinkle with cinnamon, nutmeg, 1/2 cup nuts, pressing nuts into dough. Let rise in refrigerator over night. Bake in moderate oven 18 to 20 min.

Salad Sticks

Use any roll dough desired. Roll or pat dough to 1/2 in. thickness, cut into narrow strips, brush with oil on all sides. Place 1 in. apart on greased baking sheet. Cover and let rise and bake in moderate oven 10 min.

Raised Muffins

1 cup warm water or milk
1 pkg. or cake yeast
3 tbsp. honey or blackstrap
    molasses
1 tsp. salt

3 tbsp. vegetable oil
1 cup whole wheat pastry flour
1/3 cup powdered milk
1/2 cup wheat germ flour

Dissolve yeast in water or milk and let stand while gathering other ingredients. Add honey or blackstrap, oil and salt, and stir. Sift in flour, what germ flour and powdered milk. (Wheat germ may be substituted for wheat germ flour, but of course can not be sifted. Add with flour.) Stir just enough to mix. Do not beat. Drop from tablespoon into oiled muffin pans until half full. Let rise until double in bulk. Bake at 350° for 20 min. Makes 12 large muffins.

Rye Bread #1

2 cups warm potato water
1 pkg. or cake yeast
1 tbsp. salt
1 cup mashed potatoes

4 cups rye flour
2 cups whole wheat flour
1 tsp. caraway seed

Dissolve yeast in potato water, add other ingredients, stir to mix and knead until smooth and elastic. Let rise in warm place until double in bulk. Form into loaves, place in pans, let rise. Bake at 350° to 375° one hour or longer.

Rye Bread #2

1 cup whole wheat flour
3 cups rye flour
1 tbsp. salt
Hot water

1 cake yeast
1/4 cup honey
1/4 cup lukewarm water

Mix dry ingredients. Pour in, while beating, sufficient hot water to make a stiff batter. Cover and let stand until lukewarm. Add yeast and honey dissolved in lukewarm water, and enough whole wheat flour to make a dough. Let stand until double in bulk, shape into loaves. Let rise until double in bulk. Bake at 375° one hour or longer.

Rye Bread #3

1-1/2 cups cold water
3/4 cup corn meal (yellow)
1-1/2 cups boiling water
1-1/2 tbsp. salt
1 tbsp. honey
2 cups whole wheat flour

1 pkg. or cake yeast
1/4 cup lukewarm water
1 tbsp. caraway seed
2 cups mashed potatoes
6 cups rye flour
2 tbsp. vegetable oil

Mix cornmeal with cold water in saucepan, add the boiling water, stirring constantly, and cook about 2 min. to a mush. Stir in salt, honey and oil and let cool to lukewarm. Dissolve yeast in lukewarm water, add this, the potatoes, caraway seed and flour. Mix well, knead on floured board to a smooth stiff dough. Cover and let rise in a warm place until doubled in bulk. Divide into 3 or 4 parts, shape into loaves, place in oiled pans. Let rise and bake 1 hr. at 375°.

Pumpernickel

Follow directions of above recipe, substituting rye meal for the rye flour. Make into small loaves and bake until very well done.

Quick Breads

Quick breads are usually made light with baking powder. Since double acting baking powder is made with an aluminum compound we doubt the wisdom of using it, even though it may make breads and cakes lighter and is more convenient to use. We recommend Royal Baking Powder, which is made with Cream of Tartar, a product of grapes, as its acid constituent. A mixture of Cream of Tartar and soda (2-1/2 tsp. of Cream of Tartar to 1 tsp. of soda for each quart of flour) may be used for baking powder. Since once the gas bubbles released by the combination of these have escaped from the dough or batter no more are formed, or released during cooking, breads made with this type of baking powder must be handled quickly after liquid is added and stirred as little as possible. If extra lightness is desired, more baking powder may be used, as an extra quantity of this type does not result in a bitter taste as with baking powder made with aluminum.

The elasticity of gluten is developed in breads made with wheat flour by stirring or kneading. This is desirable in yeast breads but is not necessary in quick breads and will make them less tender—another reason for handling as little as possible. Quick breads will be more tender if made from soft wheat flour which contains less gluten. Pastry flours are usually of this type. Hard wheat flour, as is used for yeast bread, may be used, however, and is probably slightly more nutritious.

Buttermilk Biscuits

2 cups whole wheat flour	1/3 cup vegetable oil
1 tsp. salt	3/4 cup buttermilk
3 tsp. Royal Baking Powder	1/4 tsp. soda

Sift dry ingredients and mix in oil. Add buttermilk all at once and stir quickly, only enough to mix. Pat out 1/2 in. thick on floured board and cut. Brush with vegetable oil and bake at 400° for 15 min.

Baking Powder Biscuits

2 cups sifted whole wheat flour	6 tbsp. vegetable oil
1 tsp. salt	2/3 cup milk
4 tsp. baking powder	

Sift dry ingredients together. Mix in oil thoroughly. Stir in milk to make a soft dough. Pat out on floured board, handling as little as possible. Cut with biscuit cutter, or in squares with knife. Bake at 375° to 400° for 15 min.

Butter may be substituted for a part of the oil in either of these recipes for better flavor, and 1/2 cup wheat germ or wheat germ flour used in place of 1/2 cup flour for extra nutrients. 1/4 cup powdered milk may be added if desired.

Drop Biscuits

Follow above recipe using 1-1/4 cup milk. Drop by spoonfuls onto oiled baking sheet or well-greased muffin tins.

Cheese Biscuits

Reduce oil to 2 tbsp. and blend in 3/4 cup sharp Cheddar cheese.

Wheat Germ Muffins

Sift together:	Mix together:
1 cup whole wheat flour	1 cup milk
1/2 tsp. salt	1/2 cup powdered milk
3 tsp. baking powder	1 egg
Add: 1-1/2 cup wheat germ	1/4 cup (each) oil and honey

Combine the two mixtures. Stir quickly and spoon into buttered muffin tins. Bake 20 min. at 400°. Makes 1 dozen large muffins. Raisins, chopped dates, or nuts may be added if desired.

Dried Fruit Muffins

2 eggs, separated
2 tbsp. oil
1 tbsp. maple syrup
1 tsp. sea kelp

1 cup figs, prunes and raisins
  chopped together
1/2 cup wheat germ
1/2 cup peanut flour

Beat the egg whites stiff and set aside. Blend the other ingredients and fold in the egg whites last. Pour batter in oiled muffin tins and bake about 25 min. at 350°. The cup of dried fruit may be of any variety, just so there is a cup of packed dried fruit after chopping. This recipe makes 6 large muffins and can be enlarged to fit the crowd. These are fine breakfast muffins.

Corn-Caraway Gems

2 eggs, separated
1 tbsp. honey
1 tsp. caraway seeds
1 tsp. sea kelp

2 tbsp. cooking oil
1/2 cup wheat germ
1/2 cup coconut or nut milk
3/4 cup yellow corn flour

Blend all ingredients except the egg whites, to be added last, beaten stiff and folded in. Bake in tiny muffin tins if possible, or in small custard cups. Have baking dishes well oiled and bake about 10 min. at 400° or until brown and done in the middle. These are crunchy and very good.

Hot Cakes

1-1/2 cup unsifted whole
  wheat flour
3 tsp. baking powder
1/2 tsp. salt

1-1/4 cup milk
1 egg
2 tbsp. honey or raw sugar
3 or 4 tbsp. oil

Sift dry ingredients together. Combine other ingredients in blender or beat eggs and then other ingredients. Combine the two mixtures, stirring just enough to mix. Bake on slightly oiled hot griddle.

Buckwheat Cakes

3/4 cup buckwheat flour
1 tsp. Royal Baking Powder
1/2 tsp. salt
1 cup milk

2 eggs, separated
1 tbsp. melted butter
1 cup cooked brown rice

Blend milk with rice, add well-beaten egg yolk. Combine dry ingredients into this mixture and add butter. Whip egg whites until stiff and fold into above mixture. Bake on oiled griddle and serve with butter and maple syrup.

Wheat Germ Pancakes

2 cups nut milk*
4 eggs, separated
2 tbsp. cooking oil
1-1/2 tsp. sea kelp

1 tsp. honey (optional)
2 cups wheat germ
1 cup brown rice flour

Beat the egg yolks, then add the milk and flour. Beat well, adding other ingredients, and fold in the stiffly beaten whites of the 4 eggs just before baking. This recipe makes about 16 nutritious pancakes.

Waffles

1 cup sifted whole wheat flour
3 tsp. baking powder
1/2 tsp. salt
2 eggs, separated

1-1/4 cups milk
1/4 cup oil
2 tsp. raw sugar

Sift dry ingredients 3 times. Add egg yolks, milk and oil, beaten together, and beat 2 min. with electric mixer on low speed. Fold in beaten egg whites and bake in preheated waffle iron.

* See Chapter VIII, Beverages

Buckwheat Waffles

2 cups water
1 tsp. lemon juice
1/4 cup raw almonds
3 tbsp. vegetable oil
Blend in blender, then add:
1/4 cup soy flour or powder

1-1/4 cups buckwheat flour
2 tbsp. honey
2 tbsp. molasses
3/4 tsp. sea salt
1/4 cup oatmeal
3/4 cup whole wheat flour

Blend thoroughly and bake in preheated waffle iron.

Nut Waffles

1 cup whole wheat flour
1/4 cup soy flour
3/4 tsp. salt
3 tsp. baking powder
1/4 to 1/2 cup chopped
pecans or other nuts

1-1/4 cups sweet milk or
almond milk*
2 eggs, separated
2 tbsp. raw sugar or honey
5 tbsp. oil

Sift dry ingredients twice. Add egg yolks, milk, sugar and oil, beaten together, and blend. Add chopped nuts and fold in egg whites.

Spicy Apple Bread

1 cup unsifted whole wheat
flour
1 tsp. soda
1 tsp. salt
1 tsp. cinnamon
1/2 tsp. nutmeg
1/2 tsp. cloves
1/2 cup butter
3/4 cup dark brown sugar

2 eggs, beaten
1 cup coarsely grated sour
apples
1 cup unsifted whole wheat
flour
1/4 cup sour milk or
buttermilk
1/2 cup chopped nuts

Sift together first six ingredients; set aside. In mixing bowl

* See Chapter VIII, Beverages

114

combine butter, sugar and eggs and beat well. Stir in apples and second cup of flour. Add sour milk and blend well; add sifted ingredients and stir just until well mixed. Add nuts and bake in greased 9x5x3 loaf pan at 350° for 55 to 60 min. Slices best after cooling for several hours or over night.

Date-Nut Bread

2 cups chopped dates	2 cups raw sugar
2 cups boiling water	4 cups sifted whole wheat flour
1 tsp. soda	1 cup chopped nuts
2 eggs	(preferably pecans)
1/2 tsp. salt	2 tsp. vanilla
2 tsp. cinnamon	3 tsp. baking powder
2 tsp. butter	

Combine boiling water and soda, then add dates and butter. Combine beaten eggs and sugar and add to first mixture. Add flour, spices, and baking powder which have been sifted together twice. Add nuts and vanilla. A cup of raisins may be added if desired. Pour into loaf pans, let stand for 5 min. Bake 1-1/4 hr. at 325° to 350°. Loaf pans should be greased and the bottom lined with waxed paper.

Nut Bread

1 cup warm potato water	2 tsp. honey
1 pkg. dry yeast	1 cup corn flour

Blend together and let rise until very light, probably around 45 min. Then add the following to make a stiff loaf:

1/2 cup sunflower seed meal	1 tbsp. oil
1 cup chopped nuts	1 cup peanut flour
1 cup raisins	1 cup wheat germ flour
1 egg, beaten	1 tsp. sea kelp

Don't bother to knead this bread because there is no gluten in it. Stir it with a big spoon, then put it into an oiled bread tin. Let it rise while the oven heats, and bake 10 min. at 400°, then about 50 min. at 350°.

Steamed Date Nut Bread

1 cup whole wheat flour	2 cups buttermilk
1 cup soy sauce	3/4 cup blackstrap molasses
1 cup wheat germ	1 tbsp. vegetable oil
3 tsp. bone meal	1 cup dates
3 tbsp. Tortula yeast	1/2 cup pecans
1-1/2 tsp. soda	

Sift together dry ingredients, except wheat germ. Add wheat germ, dates, and pecans, then other ingredients mixed together, and mix quickly, stirring as little as possible. Pour into greased molds, filling about 2/3 full, cover and steam for 2 hrs. Five #2 cans serve well as molds.

This bread is extremely high in protein, calcium, iron, and the B vitamins.

Steamed Brown Bread

1 cup all-bran	1/2 cup sugar
1 cup sour milk	1 cup whole wheat flour
1/2 cup raisins	1 tsp. soda
1 tbsp. molasses	1/4 tsp. salt

Mix all-bran, sour milk and raisins. Let it absorb the milk, then add molasses, then dry ingredients. Put into a greased coffee can (tall). Cover tightly and steam 3 hrs.

Dixie Corn Bread

4 cups soy milk	2 tbsp. cooking oil
2 cups yellow corn meal	1 tsp. sea kelp
4 eggs, separated	

Heat the milk hot, add the corn meal gradually, stirring constantly. Stir and cook until very thick. Remove from fire and cool to warm.

Beat the 4 egg whites stiff, then put the corn meal mixture, the egg yolks, oil and sea kelp under the beaters and blend them thoroughly. Fold in whites and pour the batter into an oiled oblong cake tin. Bake at 375° until done, about 45 min.

Whole Wheat Corn Meal Bread

1 cup corn meal	2/3 cup shortening
1 cup whole wheat flour	1 cup milk
2 tsp. baking powder	1 egg
1 tsp. salt	1/4 cup sugar

Combine ingredients in each of the columns above, separately, then mix or blend together and bake as in preceding recipe.

Peanut Bread

2 cups raw peanut flour	1 cup ground nuts
2 egg yolks	(preferably black walnuts)
2 rounded tbsp. homemade (or unhydrogenated) peanut butter	

Blend ingredients, adding peanut butter if too dry, or peanut flour if too sticky. Shape into thin wafers and lay them on a cooky sheet. Dry in the sun for 30 min. then store in a covered dish. These raw slices of nut bread are just delightful in flavor and high in nutrition. Made very tiny, they can be served as hors d'oeuvres. They are wonderful to munch on as between-meal snacks, or for the children's afternoon treats.

Oatmeal Crackers

1 cup cold potato water	1 tsp. sea kelp
1/2 cup cooking oil, safflower	4 cups quick-cooking oatmeal

Mix ingredients into stiff dough and chill it in refrigerator. Lightly flour a board and roll thin. Sprinkle with Seseman (sesame) seeds and roll these in. Cut in squares and bake on oiled cookie sheet at 350° for 25 min.

Whole Wheat Crackers

3 cups sifted whole wheat
   pastry flour
1/2 cup vegetable oil

1 tsp. (scant) sea salt
1/3 cup, plus 3 tbsp. soy milk

Sift flour and salt together, add oil and mix well. Add soy milk and mix to stiff dough. Roll thin, cut in desired shapes and prick with a fork. Bake at 350° until brown.

Health Crackers

2 cups whole wheat pastry
   flour
1 cup millet meal
1/2 cup rice polishings
1/4 cup sunflower seed meal

3/4 tsp. sea salt
3/4 cup vegetable oil
2 tbsp. honey
3/4 cup water

Mix dry ingredients, add oil and blend in well with fingers or pastry cutter. Add honey dissolved in water, mix and knead very lightly. Roll to thickness of piecrust. Cut into squares and prick with fork. Bake at 350° until brown.

Cereals

Whole Wheat

1 cup clean whole wheat
1 tsp. salt

2 cups water

Bring water to a boil and add salt and wheat. Remove from direct heat as soon as water reaches second boil, pour in casserole dish and place, uncovered, on adapter ring or shelf of steamer or deep well cooker. Have boiling water in bottom of steamer to within 1 in. of shelf. Cover steamer tightly, and cook over low heat to keep water in steamer just simmering for 8 to 10 hrs. Serve with butter or cream and honey.

Cracked Wheat

1 cup cracked wheat   1 tsp. salt
4 cups water

Add salt and cracked wheat to boiling water and cook over direct heat for about 30 min. or in double boiler for 1 hr. or more. This may be started in double boiler at night and cooked for 30 min. then finished cooking in the morning.

Another method of cooking, which would retain more of the vitamins but perhaps make the wheat less easily digested, is as follows:
Add 1 cup cracked wheat to 3 cups boiling salted water. Boil for 5 min. then put into quart thermos to retain heat and leave for 8 hrs. before serving.

Multi-Grain Dry Cereal

3 cups whole wheat flour   1-1/2 cups dry malt
3 cups corn meal   3-1/2 cups milk or soy milk
3 cups millet flour   4 tbsp. honey
3 cups oatmeal   1 tbsp. salt or sea salt

Blend dry ingredients together. Mix milk, malt and honey and add to dry ingredients to make a stiff dough. Roll very thin, prick, and bake at 300° until golden brown. Put through food chopper to crumble it.

Dry Cereal #2

1 cup whole wheat flour
1/2 cup rye flour
1 cup soy flour
1/2 cup corn meal
1 cup oatmeal
1/2 cup rice bran

1 tbsp. sea salt
1/2 cup water
1/2 cup honey
1/2 cup oil
3 tsp. toasted sesame seeds

Mix dry ingredients. Add water, honey and oil mixed together, and stir to form granules. Bake on a sheet pan at 325° until lightly browned, stirring frequently. Turn out fire, and allow to stay in oven, stirring occasionally until cool. How long your oven retains enough heat to cook will determine the degree of brownness before fire is turned off.

CHAPTER 7: DESSERTS AND SWEETS

While we can find no corroboration from scientific sources of the statement in the Cayce readings that beet sugar is preferable to cane sugar (or, in fact, that there is any difference, from a chemical standpoint), the deleterious effects of refined sugars and an excess of concentrated sweets are widely recognized.

According to Adelle Davis, one of the country's best known nutritionists,* excessive eating of sweets, especially refined sugar, increases the need for choline, a deficiency of which has been found to produce nephritis and liver damage, and interferes with the absorption of calcium by increasing the production of alkaline digestive juices, thus counteracting the acidity of the digestive juices of the stomach necessary to dissolve calcium. She also notes that persons suffering from antherosclerosis often show a particularly high intake of refined sugar.

J.I. Rodale, Editor of *Prevention Magazine,* relates the consumption of refined sugars to susceptibility to insect bites, sinus trouble, stomach trouble, arthritis, pyorrhea, dental decay and cancer. He stresses the price we pay in vitamin B for eating refined sugar, stating that B vitamins, occurring in the natural sweets, fruits, and sugar cane, are necessary for the assimilation of sugars, and when refined sugars are eaten these vitamins are drawn from the organs and tissues of the body, leaving them deficient in these important food substances.

The relation of sugar consumption to dental decay is generally recognized. In an article in the *Journal of the American Dental Association* for July 1, 1947, Isaac Schour,

* Let's Eat Right to Keep Fit"
"Let's Get Well—Harcourt, Brace and World, Inc., N.Y.

D.D.S., Ph.D., and Maury Massler, D.D.S., M.S., in discussing the low incidence of tooth decay among children of post-war Italy, as compared to the enormously higher rate (several times as high) among children of the same ages in this country, point out that the diet of the Italian children included very little refined sugar, although it was high in starches and the children were not especially well nourished.

Melvin Page, D.D.S., in his book, "Degeneration—Regeneration," states that sugar is indirectly a cause of dental decay, pyorrhea and arthritis by disturbing the calcium-phosphorus balance. Sugar disturbs this balance, he says, more than any other single factor. The amounts of these materials, he believes, is not as important as their proportions to each other. He also states that he does not remember seeing a single cancer case that showed correct sugar level of the blood.

Michael H. Walsh, M.Sc., F.R.I.C., Instructor of Clinical Nutrition at the University of California, stated in a speech in April, 1950,* that there is evidence of a dietary relationship between high sugar consumption and polio, rheumatic fever, arthritis and many degenerative diseases.

According to J. I. Rodale,[1] Dr. Sandler brought to a standstill a polio epidemic in North Carolina several years ago, by means of a diet the essence of which was a sharp reduction in the consumption of sugar. Apparently large numbers of residents were sufficiently frightened by the proportions of the epidemic to be willing to try the diet he recommended. His theory was that low blood sugar, brought about by eating too much sugar and thus triggering an overproduction of insulin, can increase the susceptibility to polio.

Dr. E. M. Abrahamson, in his book, "Body, Mind and Sugar," not only agrees with Dr. Sandler, but relates low blood sugar to such a wide variety of ills as asthma, alcoholism, neuroses, fatigue, rheumatic fever, ulcers, epilepsy, depression, and so forth, and explains how consumption of concentrated sweets produces low blood sugar through stimulating the pancreas to excessive production of insulin.

* "Sugar and Dental Caries"—*Journal of the California State Dental Association, 1950*
[1] "The Health Finder"—The Rodale Press, 123 New Bond St., London

All sweets, save natural sweets such as found in most fruits, maple syrups, and honey, are acid producing, another reason why the consumption of them should be strictly limited. Fruits (fresh, stewed or dried), confections and desserts made with dried fruits and honey as the only sweetening agent, and honey used on bread and cereals, can supply the sugars necessary to form the alcohol needed for a proper digestion and assimilation, and are most to be recommended from a nutritional standpoint, although an excess even of these can produce an unhealthy imbalance.

Raw sugar was among those sweets recommended by the Cayce readings. Real raw sugar, we have been told (that is, sugar which has not gone through the refining process), is now impractical to obtain in this country. That which is sold as raw sugar at the present time is produced by adding molasses to refined white sugar, thereby replacing the vitamins and minerals which have been removed in the refining process.

Whether factors as yet unknown have been altered by this process, making this inferior to real raw sugar, we have no way of knowing, but it is certainly preferable to cane sugar without the addition of the mineral-rich molasses. Therefore, since most people will eat some cookies, cakes, puddings, and such, we have included here some recipes for these, which use raw sugar and other natural sweets. However, we would remind the reader of the warning in the readings against the combination of starches and sweets.

Protein Cake

1/2 lb. nut meats, ground fine	1 cup raw or brown sugar or
7 eggs, separated	1/2 of each
Pinch of salt	1 tsp. vanilla

Beat egg whites until very stiff and dry. Set aside. Beat egg yolks and sugar together until creamy, add nut meats gradually, then salt and vanilla. Fold this mixture into the egg whites carefully, and bake in an ungreased tube pan for 1 hr. at 325°. Invert pan to cool.

Caramel Sauce

2/3 cup maple syrup   4 tbsp. cream
2/3 cup brown sugar

Simmer a couple of minutes, partly cool, and add 1 tbsp. butter; finish cooling.

Carob Cake

1/2 cup butter   1-1/2 tsp. cinnamon
1 cup raw sugar   1/2 tsp. baking powder
2 eggs   1/2 tsp. baking soda
1 cup sifted whole wheat pastry 1/2 tsp. salt
   flour   1/2 cup buttermilk
1/2 cup carob powder   1 tsp. vanilla

Cream butter and sugar. Add eggs and beat well. Combine all dry ingredients and sift together three times. Add sifted dry ingredients to creamed mixture, alternating with buttermilk, beating well. Pour into an oiled 8x8 baking pan. Bake at 350° for 25-30 min. Frost with Carob Fudge Frosting.

Carob Fudge Frosting

3/4 cup rich milk   1/4 cup butter
1/4 cup carob powder   2 cups raw sugar

Place first three ingredients in saucepan over medium heat, stir constantly until smooth and thick. Add sugar and stir until completely dissolved. Without stirring, cook until the "soft ball" stage when tested in cold water. Frost cooled cake.

Oatmeal Cake

1 cup oatmeal	2 eggs
1/2 cup chopped dates or raisins	1 tsp. vanilla
	1/2 tsp. salt
1/2 cup butter	1 tsp. baking soda
2 cups brown sugar	1-1/2 cups whole wheat flour

Pour 1/2 cup boiling water over oatmeal and fruit. Stir well and cool. After it is cooled, mix and add remaining ingredients to oatmeal and fruit mixture. Bake at 375° for 30 min.

Topping

1/2 cup brown sugar	2 tbsp. water
1/4 cup whole wheat flour	3/4 cup nuts or coconut
1/4 cup butter	

Melt butter, add water, flour, sugar and coconut. Spread over cake and return to oven for about 10 min.

Deluxe Spice Cup Cakes

1 cup uncooked prunes or dates, pitted and chopped (may substitute 2 cans of thick applesauce)	1 tsp. salt
	1-1/4 tsp. soda
	1 tsp. each: cinnamon, nutmeg, cloves, ginger, allspice
1 cup boiling water	3 eggs
2 cups unsifted whole wheat flour	1 cup raisins (optional)
	1/2 cup vegetable oil
1-1/2 cups dark brown sugar	

Pour cup of boiling water over dried fruit. Let stand at a minimum of 2 hrs. (omit this step if using applesauce.) Place fruit mixture and all other ingredients (except raisins) in small bowl of mixer. Blend for 1 min. on low speed. Beat 2 min. on medium speed. Add raisins. Stir in. Makes 2 dozen medium cup cakes. (Use liners). Bake 25 min. at 350°. When cold, sift over top of cakes, 1 part dried milk to 1 part powdered sugar.

Peanut Cookies

1 cup chopped organically grown peanuts	1/2 cup homemade (or unhydrogenated) peanut butter
1-1/2 cups peanut flour	

Mix the ingredients together. If too dry, add drops of salad oil. If too sticky, add soy milk powder. Shape into small cookies and roll in sunflower seed meal. Store in the refrigerator. These cookies satisfy the peanut lover's taste for peanuts, and are easily digested. Even the children and aged can eat them safely and they are a high protein dessert or snack.

Nutty Confections

Put 1/4 lb. of brick carob to melt. Meanwhile, chop the following ingredients and form the mixture into thin cookies:

1 cup locally grown nuts	1-1/2 cups pitted dates, chopped
1 cup shelled peanuts	1 cup grated coconut
1/2 cup sunflower seeds	

Dip the thin cookies into the warm carob mixture, on both sides, then lay on an oiled pan until the carob is reset. Serve as cookies.

Health Cookies

2 cups raw sugar (yellow D)	3-1/2 cups whole wheat flour
1/2 lb. (2 sticks) butter, softened	2 tsp. soda
3 eggs	1-1/2 tsp. cream of tartar
2 cups coconut, fine, unsweetened	1 cup sunflower seeds, shelled

Cream together sugar, butter, and eggs. Add coconut. Blend. Combine flour, soda and cream of tartar, and add to first mixture, mix, and add sunflower seeds. Let stand 1 hr. in refrigerator, if possible, as the mixture is then easier to handle. Pinch off teaspoonfuls and flatten almost to paper thin, using a wet cloth over a flat-bottom jar or wide glass. Bake at 375° about 7-8 min. Makes about 75 cookies.

Fig Fandangos

3 eggs, separated	1 tsp. sea kelp
2/3 cup honey	1/2 tsp. cinnamon
1 tsp. pure vanilla extract	1 cup peanut flour
1 cup nut meats, chopped	1/2 cup wheat germ flour
1 cup figs, chopped	

Beat the egg whites and set aside. Blend the other items and fold the egg whites in last. Bake in a 9x9-in. tin about 45 min. at 350°. Try with a toothpick, making sure it is done before removing from oven. Cool and cut in squares. This is very light; take out with a pancake turner or slanting spatula.

Coconut Macaroons

1/2 cup raw sugar	1/8 tsp. salt
2 egg whites	1/2 tsp. vanilla
1/2 tsp. cider vinegar	1/2 cup coconut, shredded

Beat whites until foamy, then add vinegar and salt. Beat until peaks hold, gradually add sugar, a tablespoon at a time, beating well after each addition. Lightly fold in vanilla and coconut. Drop by tablespoon on brown paper or cookie sheet. Sprinkle top of cookies with coconut. Bake at 275.°

Uncooked Taffy

1/2 cup homemade (or unhydrogenated) peanut butter	1 cup peanuts—shelled from whole unroasted peanuts
1/2 cup honey	Instant soy milk powder

Blend the first three ingredients together (the peanuts may be chopped if desired). Then use only enough of the soy milk powder to make a stiff dough. Roll it in a long roll, place on a cookie sheet, and chill over night. In the morning, whack off inch pieces for the lunch pail, or for the children for special treats.

Lollipops

1 cup raisins
1 cup dried prunes
1 cup locally grown nut meats

1 cup coconut chunks
1 cup figs

Put the above ingredients through the food grinder and shape into balls, then flatten into oblongs. Roll each one in either ground coconut meal, ground nuts, or ground sunflower seeds, and put a wooden paddle in each lollipop. A treat for the children.

Date Carob Bars

4 eggs, separated, whites beaten stiff
1/3 cup honey
3/4 cup dates, pitted and chopped

3/4 cup almonds, ground
3/4 cup wheat germ
1/3 cup carob powder

Blend egg yolks with other ingredients, fold in the whites last and bake in a small cake tin about 45 min. at about 325°, or until done. Cut in bars while warm.
This recipe may be varied by changing the fruit and nuts and by adding different spices with the various combinations.

Candy

1 cup "Grandma's Molasses"
1 tbsp. butter

1 cup raw sugar

Cook slowly for 10 min. (270° candy thermometer) and pull until candy becomes light in color.

Dried Fruits and Nuts

Date Patties

Press 1 cup dates and 1 cup pecans through food chopper, mix thoroughly. Form into patties and roll in coconut or Malba nuts.

Natural Candy Bars

Press 1 lb. black Mission figs with 2 cups almonds through food chopper. Roll out 1/2 in. thickness on wax paper to prevent sticking to board. Cut in bars 3 in. long and 1 in. wide. Cover each bar with Mal-ba nuts and wrap in wax paper.

Raisin Balls

Raisins ground and formed into balls and rolled in freshly grated coconut.

Fig Candy

Take desired number of white figs, cut off 3/4 in. of stem end and open fig for stuffing. Put equal parts of fresh coconut and sesame seeds through food chopper. Add a little Mal-ba nuts and stuff each fig fully. Garnish each fig with a pine nut.

Carrot Pudding

1/2 cup butter	2 tbsp. lemon peel, finely
3/4 cup brown sugar	chopped
1 egg	1-1/4 cups whole wheat flour,
2 tbsp. water	1 tsp. baking powder
3/4 cup raw carrots, grated	1/2 tsp. salt
1/3 cup dates, chopped	1/3 tsp. cinnamon
1/2 cup seedless raisins	1/2 tsp. nutmeg
1/2 cup nuts, chopped	1/8 tsp. allspice

Cream together butter and sugar until light and fluffy, add egg and water and beat thoroughly. Add carrots, dates, raisins, nuts, and lemon peel, blend well. Sift together flour, baking powder, salt, cinnamon, nutmeg and allspice, and gradually add to creamed mixture. Turn into buttered 5-cup mold.

Bake for 1-1/4 to 1-1/2 hrs. at 325.° Allow to stand for 5 min. Remove from mold. Serve warm. Serves 8 to 10. Pudding may be prepared ahead of time and refrigerated or frozen. To reheat, wrap in foil and place in oven until heated through.

Fruit Crumb Pudding

Mix 1 pt. whole wheat crumbs in pt. hot milk and let stand for 10 min. Steam 1-1/2 cups mixed raisins, dates, and figs for 5 min. Add to bread crumbs. Then add 1 egg, beaten. Mix thoroughly and bake for 30 min.

Date Cream

1 cup dates, pitted	1-1/2 cup whipped cream
1 cup applesauce	

Mash dates and mix with applesauce to which add whipped cream. Pile into sherbet glasses and chill.

Date Coconut Cream

1 cup dates, pitted and ground   2 cups whipped cream
1/2 cup fresh coconut

Combine ingredients and chill thoroughly.

Vanilla Rice Custard

3 tbsp. natural brown rice,   3 tbsp. dark brown sugar
  unpolished   1 tsp. vanilla
1 cup milk, skim or whole   1/2 cup raisins (optional)
1 egg, beaten slightly

Nutmeg to sprinkle over top when ingredients are well mixed.
Bake in 325° oven for about 1 hr. or until silver knife comes
out clean after testing.

Coconut Custard

3 eggs, beaten   2 cups coconut milk
1/3 cup honey   1/4 tsp. mace
1 tsp. pure vanilla

Beat well and pour into a small baking dish. Set this in a pan
of hot water and bake until the custard is set in the center.
Cool, then grate fresh coconut over the top and serve.

Coconut Rice

1 cup boiling hot brown rice   1/2 cup almonds, chopped
1 egg yolk   1/2 cup coconut milk
1 tsp. honey
1/2 cup fresh-shredded
  coconut

Blend these ingredients and stir into the boiling rice, then
remove from the fire and cool.

131

Glorified Rice

1 cup brown rice, cooked
1 cup crushed pineapple,
   drained

1/3 cup honey
1/2 tsp. salt
1 cup whipped cream

Mix ingredients, and fold in whipped cream.

Dried Apricots in Gelatin

3/4 cup dried apricots
1 pkg. (small) peach gelatin
1/4 cup yogurt

Hot water to cover apricots
1 cup boiling water to
   dissolve gelatin

Allow apricots to soak and cool a few hours or over night.
Purée in blender and add peach gelatin made with only 1 cup
water. Put 1/2 mixture from blender in bowl or mold and let
stand until it sets—10 min.—then either mix in the yogurt or
spread it on top of mixture in bowl. Then cover with remaining blender mixture.

Lemon Cream Gelatin Dessert or Salad

1pkg. gelatin. Sweeten and flavor with 1 cup natural sugar and
the juice of 1 lemon (about 2 tbsp. lemon juice)
1 cup crushed unsweetened pineapple, drained
2 cups hot water (Use the juice drained from the pineapple and
also count the liquid from the lemon to amount to a portion of
the liquid, then add enough hot water to make up to the 2
cups.)
1/2 cup Cheddar cheese,   1/2 pt. whipping cream
   grated

Dissolve the gelatin. Add all the liquid. Chill until just set.
Then add the crushed pineapple, grated cheese, and fold in
the whipped cream. Serves 4 to 6.

Strawberry Ice

2 cups fresh hulled strawberries 1/2 cup honey
2 egg yolks 1 cup fresh pineapple juice

Put all the above in a blender. (If you have no fresh raw pineapple juice, use a heaping tablespoon of chopped raw pineapple and 3/4 cup cold water.) Pour this mixture into a freezing-tray and stir it several times while it freezes.

Honey Freeze

6 eggs, separated 1 envelope unflavored gelatin
1/2 tsp. salt Whipped cream
1-1/2 cups honey Pistachio nuts, chopped

Beat egg yolks until thick and lemon colored. Combine with salt, honey and gelatin in the top of a double boiler. Cook over boiling water, stirring constantly, until mixture is somewhat thickened and smooth. Cool mixture in a pan of ice water until thoroughly chilled. Beat egg whites until soft peaks form. Gently fold egg yolk mixture into egg whites. Pour mixture into freezer trays or individual molds. Freeze 2 hrs. Serve with garnish of whipped cream and nuts. Makes about 1-1/2 qts.

French Strawberry Pie

2 baskets strawberries 3-1/2 tbsp. corn starch
1 (3 oz.) pkg. cream cheese 1 tbsp. lemon juice
1 baked pie shell 1/3 cup whipping cream
1-1/4 cups sugar, unrefined

Spread softened cream cheese in bottom of pie shell and press 1/2 of the choicest berries whole into the cheese, tips up.

Mash remaining berries. Measure to make 1-1/2 cups berries and juice (add water if necessary). Mix corn starch and sugar. Add berries and lemon juice and cook until thick. Add a few drops food coloring and cool. Pour over pie shell containing creamed cheese and strawberries. Chill 4 hrs. Serve garnished with whipping cream.

CHAPTER 8: BEVERAGES

Milk was frequently recommended in the readings, especially certified raw milk. The use of raw milk is contrary to opinions stated in many health magazines and books, but most nutritionists recognize the nutritional importance of milk itself as the most nearly complete single food known. Soy and nut milk recipes are included here, primarily for the benefit of those who may be allergic to cow's milk, since these furnish most of the nutritional elements of the natural milk.

Since chocolate is now deemed generally detrimental to health, recipes are given using carob, a chocolate substitute, and other ingredients both pleasing to the taste and healthful from the viewpoint of the readings.

Raw vegetable juices have most of the nutritional value of the vegetables from which they are prepared and can be taken in much larger quantities than would be possible with the whole vegetable. Since roughage is important in the diet we suggest adding these, rather than substituting juice for the raw fresh vegetables. One individual was advised by the readings to take vegetable juices, either separately or in combination, once or twice a week. (1709-10) Another was told to take an ounce of raw carrot juice at least once a day. Vegetable juices may be obtained at health food stores, or can be prepared at home with a vegetable juicer.

Fruit juices as beverages, likewise, add more of the values of fresh fruit to the diet, but should not be substituted for fresh fruit. Citrus fruit juices were those most often recommended in the readings, and it was suggested that lime or lemon juice be added to orange or grapefruit juice; (2072-3), (3525-1) also that lemon and lime juice be combined.

Milk Drinks

Carob Milk Drink #1

2 cups certified raw milk
2 tbsp. carob powder

2 tbsp. honey
1/4 cup water

Heat milk, don't boil, and pour over remaining ingredients.

Carob Milk Drink #2

1 small carob candy bar   2 cups certified raw milk

Melt carob candy in top of double boiler, add milk and warm to desired temperature. Don't boil. Sweeten with honey, if desired.

Carrot Milk

1 cup certified raw milk
2 med. size carrots, cut in
   pieces

Place ingredients in blender and liquefy. This drink has an attractive pale-carrot tint and a coconut-like flavor.

Apricot Milk

1 cup ripe raw apricots or
1/2 cup cooked dried apricots

3 cups certified raw milk
Honey to taste

Place ingredients in blender and liquefy.

Maple-Egg Milk

3 tbsp. pure maple syrup   1/4 tsp. pure vanilla
1 egg yolk   Dash of salt
2 cups certified raw milk

Blend ingredients 15 to 20 sec.

Yogurt (Bulgarian Buttermilk)

Bulgarian buttermilk, recommended by the Cayce readings, and more commonly known in this country as yogurt, has been one of the principal foods of the Bulgarians for a long period of time, and is considered by many to be largely responsible for their unusual health, vigor and virility. The 1930 census showed that there were more than 1600 Bulgarians over 100 years old per million of population, compared with only 9 persons in America. Baldness and white hair are said to be almost unknown in Bulgaria.

The health-giving properties of yogurt are primarily due to the fact that the bacteria in yogurt, Lactobacillus bulgarius, streptococcus lactis, thermobacterium yogurt, thrive in the intestines and are capable of synthesizing large amounts of the entire group of B vitamins, as well as destroying or inhibiting the action of putrefactive bacteria. The bacteria also partially break down the proteins of the milk, making it more easy to digest, and the acid produced in the milk dissolves some of the calcium, making it more available to the body.

Yogurt may be beaten and served as a beverage, having a flavor very similar to buttermilk. If the taste is not enjoyed at first, as is frequently the case, a taste for it may be cultivated gradually by taking it frequently in very small amounts. It may also be served with fruit or berries or as an ingredient in salad dressings.

Preparing Yogurt at Home

Basic recipe: Combine 1 quart pasteurized whole or skim milk and 1/4 cup commercial yogurt. Warm slowly in oven or top of double boiler or in glasses set in a pan of warm water over simmer burner until milk reaches temperature of 100° to 120°. Maintain at temperature between 90° and 120 until milk becomes the consistency of junket, or from 3 to 5 hrs. If temperature is kept lower than 90° lactic acid bacteria, rather than the yogurt culture, will grow; and while these will thicken the milk and are not harmful, they cannot live in the intestinal tract to produce B vitamins. If temperature rises above 120° the bacteria will be killed and milk will not thicken.

Thick yogurt: Combine 3 cups pasteurized milk, 1-1/2 cups evaporated milk and 1/4 cup commercial yogurt, or combine 1 quart pasteurized milk, 1 cup powdered skim milk, and 1/4 cup yogurt. Proceed as above.

If raw milk is used instead of pasteurized, heat to simmering and cool to 120° before adding yogurt starter.
As soon as yogurt has thickened to custard consistency, it should be refrigerated, and may be kept for several days. 1/4 cup of this home-made yogurt may be used to start the next batch instead of commercial yogurt. Yogurt culture may be used, instead, as a starter. It can be obtained from International Yogurt Co., 8478 Melrose Place, Los Angeles 46, California.

Grape Buttermilk (or Yogurt) Drink

1/4 cup grape juice	2 tbsp. honey
2 tbsp. lemon juice	
1 pt. Bulgarian buttermilk or yogurt	

Blend about 15 sec.

Buttermilk (or Yogurt) Drink

2 tbsp. honey
1 egg
1 pt. Bulgarian buttermilk, or
  yogurt

1 tbsp. lemon juice
1/2 tsp. lemon rind, grated

Blend for about 20 sec.

Orange Buttermilk (or Yogurt) Drink

1/2 cup orange juice
1-1/2 cups Bulgarian
  buttermilk or yogurt

2 tbsp. honey
1/2 tsp. orange rind, grated

Blend about 20 sec. Delicious, even for those who do not care for buttermilk or yogurt.

Pineapple Buttermilk (or Yogurt)

1 cup Bulgarian buttermilk (or
  yogurt)
1/2 cup pineapple juice,
  unsweetened

1/2 cup fresh papaya, diced

Place all ingredients in blender, and blend until papaya is liquefied.

BABY FORMULAS

Evaporated Milk (Newborn)

Carnation evaporated milk,
  10 oz.

Water, 20 oz.
Unpasteurized honey, 2 tbsp.

This will make 30 oz. of formula, which will probably be more than the average newborn will need in 24 hrs., until he weighs 9 or 10 lbs.

Full Strength Formula, Evaporated Milk

Carnation evaporated milk,
  13 oz.

Water, 19 oz.
Unpasteurized honey, 3 tbsp.

This will make about 5-1/4 oz. in 6 bottles; 6-1/2 oz. in 5 bottles; 8 oz. in 4 bottles.

Raw Milk Formula (Newborn)

Certified raw milk, preferably goat milk, 15 oz.; unpasteurized honey, 3 tbsp. : "Mineral Cocktail" water (see below), 15 oz.

This will make 30 oz. of formula. When the child is 2 or 3 months, half the quantity of water would be sufficient for the dilution of the milk. After 3 months, the milk can be taken straight.

"Mineral Cocktail"

Boil Irish potato skins in water (used above) for about 15-20 min.

Soy Milk made from Soya Powder

1 cup soya powder
4 cups cold water
1 tbsp. honey

1 tsp. liquid lecithin or
  1 tbsp. salad oil
1/4 tsp. salt

Liquefy the soya powder in cold water. Let stand for 2 hrs. Then cook over double boiler for 1 hr. When cool, add to other ingredients. This milk is very rich and may be liquefied with seed milks for a wholesome palatable milk: 1 cup soy milk to 1 cup almond, cashew, etc. nut milk.

Soy Milk made from Soy Flour

1 cup soy flour
2 cups water
1/4 cup honey

1 tbsp. liquid lecithin, or
    1/4 cup salad oil
1/2 tsp. salt

Liquefy the soy flour and water and cook in double boiler for 1 hr. When cool, liquefy again with the remaining ingredients. Pour the oil in gradually, while other ingredients are blending. Add enough water to make 2-1/2 qts. of liquid. This milk may be used in any recipe calling for liquid soy milk.

Soy Bean Milk made from Whole Soy Beans

Soak 1 cup raw soy beans for 3 days in the refrigerator, pouring water off each day and adding fresh water. On the 3rd day, pour off water and liquefy the beans with 4-5 cups fresh water. Extract all milk, by running liquefied beans through a juice press, a fine strainer or cloth bag. Put the milk in double boiler and cook for 1 hr. Liquefy again.

Carob Shake

2 cups soy milk
  (see previous recipe)
2 rounded tbsp. carob powder
2 tbsp. honey

5 pitted dates
4 rounded tbsp. raw almond or
  cashew butter
2 tbsp. pure vanilla

Liquefy ingredients together. Chill and liquefy again.

Almond Milk

(Basic Nut Milk Recipe)

1/2 cup blanched almonds
2 cups water
Honey to taste

Salt to taste
1 tsp. liquid lecithin

Liquefy nuts and water, add remaining ingredients. Almonds are a perfect protein food. This recipe may be used for raw peanuts, pine nuts, sunflower seeds, sesame seeds, brazil and hazel nuts, pecans, etc.

Carob and Nut Milk Drink

1/2 cup raw cashews, or almonds	1/4 cup water
	2 tbsp. honey
2 cups water	2 tbsp. carob powder

Liquefy the nuts with the 2 cups of water. Heat, but do not boil the milk. Pour the milk over mixture of remaining ingredients, stirring until blended.

Fruit and Vegetable Beverages

Pineapple-Watercress Cocktail

2 cups pineapple juice	1 thick slice peeled lemon or
1 bunch watercress, washed	2 tbsp. lemon juice
3 tbsp. honey	1 cup cracked ice

Blend until cress is reduced to drinkability. Serves 4.

Vegetable Cocktail

2 cups tomato juice	1 slice green pepper
1 small stalk celery, with leaves, cut up	1 slice onion
	1/4 tsp. salt
2 or 3 sprigs parsley	1/2 tsp. honey
2 slices lemon, with peel	1 cup cracked ice

Blend until vegetables are completely liquefied. Serves 4-5.

Pineapple & Alfalfa-Sprouts Drink

2 cups unsweetened pineapple
juice or orange juice
1 cup alfalfa sprouts

2 tbsp. almond butter
Honey to taste

Place ingredients in blender and liquefy.

Cranberry Cocktail

2 cups raw cranberries,
unsprayed
1 cup water
1 cup orange juice

1/2 cup honey
Dash of salt
Juice of 1 lime

Blend until liquefied. Strain and chill before serving.

Orange-Coconut Drink

1-1/2 cups shredded coconut
3 cups water
1 can frozen orange juice

Juice of 1 lime
1 cup cracked ice

Simmer coconut and water for 10 min. Cool, strain and add
remaining ingredients. Blend about 15 sec. Pour over more
cracked ice in tall glasses.

Raspberry Punch

1-1/2 cups raspberry juice
1/4 cup lemon juice
1 cup orange juice
1/4 cup lime juice

1/2 cup honey
1/2 small cucumber, diced
1 qt. water

Blend all ingredients, except water, until cucumber is liquefied.
Let stand in refrigerator several hrs. Strain and add water.

Fruit and Vegetable Juice Combinations (1 pint)

Celery juice ....10 oz.	Celery juice .... 7 oz.
Spinach juice .... 4 oz.	Lettuce juice .... 5 oz.
Parsley juice .... 2 oz.	Spinach juice .... 4 oz.
Carrot juice ....11 oz.	Carrot juice ....13 oz.
Coconut juice .... 2 oz.	Coconut juice .... 3 oz.
Beet juice .... 3 oz.	
	Carrot juice .... 9 oz.
	Beet juice .... 3 oz.
Carrot juice ....10 oz.	Lettuce juice .... 4 oz.
Beet juice .... 3 oz.	
Spinach juice .... 3 oz.	Carrot juice .... 7 oz.
	Celery juice .... 4 oz.
Carrot juice ....10 oz.	Parsley juice .... 2 oz.
Spinach juice .... 3 oz.	Spinach juice .... 3 oz.
Mustard greens juice ...... 3 oz.	
	Carrot juice .... 9 oz.
Carrot juice .... 7 oz.	Celery juice .... 5 oz.
Celery juice .... 5 oz.	Endive juice .... 2 oz.
Lettuce juice .... 4 oz.	
	Cucumber juice .... 3 oz.
Cucumber juice .... 6 oz.	Watercress juice .... 3 oz.
Radish juice .... 5 oz.	Celery juice .... 3 oz.
Green pepper juice .... 5 oz.	Tomato juice .... 4 oz.
	Parsley juice .... 3 oz.
Coconut milk .... 8 oz.	
Fig juice .... 8 oz.	Orange juice .... 7 oz.
	Lime juice .... 1 oz.
Dandelion greens juice ... 8 oz.	Pomegranate juice .... 8 oz.
Pineapple juice .... 8 oz.	4 egg yolks
	Honey ....4 tsp.
Pineapple juice .... 8 oz.	
Cabbage juice .... 8 oz.	Strawberry juice .... 5 oz.
Almond butter ....4 tsp.	Rhubarb juice .... 5 oz.
	Pineapple juice .... 6 oz.
Orange juice .... 8 oz.	
Lime juice .... 1 oz.	Grapefruit juice .... 8 oz.
Celery juice .... 7 oz.	Lemon juice .... 1 oz.
Almond butter ....4 tsp.	Spinach juice .... 3 oz.
	Pineapple juice .... 4 oz.

144

Boysenberry-Coconut Drink

1-1/2 cups boysenberry juice
3/4 cup coconut juice
1/2 cup orange juice

1 tsp. lime juice
2 tbsp. honey

Liquefy together.

Prune-Coconut Drink

1-1/2 cups prune juice
1/2 cup orange juice

1 tsp. lime juice
1 cup fresh coconut juice

Liquefy together.

CHAPTER 9: SOUPS AND BROTHS

It is not difficult to understand, from a nutritional standpoint, why soups and broths were recommended in the readings in almost every case where advice was given concerning the menu. They are easily digested and when properly prepared contain an abundance of minerals and vitamins in easily assimilated form. The readings particularly recommended broths of the bony pieces of fowl for their calcium content, (808-15) and vegetable soups carrying the marrow of beef bones, (1523-8). Gelatin, which is needed to enable the body to utilize vitamins, (849-75) is also extracted by boiling bones for stock. Vegetable parings boiled along with the bones add extra important minerals to the stock and fresh vegetables may be utilized in soups with little loss of vitamins or minerals.

In making soup stock, bones having bits of meat clinging to them should be browned slowly to develop a more enjoyable flavor, then boiled for 3 to 4 hrs. or cooked in water in a pressure cooker for 1/2 hr. or longer. Since it is desirable to break down the connective tissue as much as possible, thereby extracting the greatest possible amount of gelatin and calcium, cooking at high temperatures is preferable to simmering. Adding a small amount of vinegar also hastens the breakdown of connective tissue and increases the amount of calcium and gelatin obtained. The calcium combines with and counteracts the acid. Salt should be added with the water, as this aids in drawing out the juices in the scraps of meat and bones. Vegetable parings should be added only during the last 15 min. of cooking, and vegetables (added after straining the stock to remove bones and parings) should be finely chopped and cooked quickly in the stock, only as long as necessary for tenderness.

146

The following recipe for Beef Juice was given in reading 1343-2 and advised for several people receiving readings. It was referred to "as medicine" (5374-1) or "almost as medicine" (1100-10). Instructions for eating were explicit:

Take at least a tablespoon during a day, or two table-spoonfuls. But not as spoonfuls, rather sips of same. This sipped, in this manner, will work towards producing the gastric flow through the intestinal system.   1100-10

Pure Beef Juice

Take a pound to a pound and a half of beef, preferably of the round steak. No fat and no portions other than that which is of the muscle or tendon for strength; no fatty or skin portions. Dice this into half-inch cubes, as it were, or practically so. Put same in a glass jar without water . . . Put the jar into a boiler or container with the water coming to about half or three-fourths toward the top of the jar. Put a cloth in the container to prevent the jar from cracking. Do not seal the jar tight, but cover the top. Let this boil (the water, with the jar in same) for 3 to 4 hrs.

Then strain off the juice. The refuse may be pressed somewhat. It will be found that the meat or flesh itself will be worthless. Place the juice in a cool place, but do not keep too long; never longer than 3 days. Hence the quantity made up at the time depends upon how much or how often the body will take this.   1343-2

Soups

Delightful, nutritious soups may be made by adding cooked natural brown unpolished rice to chicken broth, beef broth or bouillon cubes with fine slivered onions. Just before serving add toasted, buttered croutons.

Chicken Soup with Rice or Noodles

1-3/4 lb. stewing chicken cut
  into quarters
1 carrot
2 qts. cold water
1 stalk celery
1 med. onion

2 tsp. salt
1/4 tsp. pepper
1/4 cup uncooked brown rice
  or whole wheat noodles
2 tbsp. parsley, minced

Place chicken, carrot, water, celery, onion, salt and pepper in a 4-1/2 qt. pot. Cover and simmer approx. 2 hrs., or until meat is tender. Remove chicken from pot, strain the liquid and remove all possible fat. Return the stock to pot, bring to boil, add rice or noodles, cover and cook until tender. Add parsley. Serves 4-6.

Chicken Soup

2 cups chicken broth
1 cup chicken meat
1 small can tomatoes
1/2 pkg. frozen peas or
  leftovers

4 stalks celery, diced
1 cup cashews, raw
Dash salt

Boil bony pieces of chicken in water to cover, to which 1 medium size onion has been added. When chicken is tender, remove from heat, cool and remove meat from bones.
Place first 5 ingredients in blender, blending well. Add more broth, if desired. Place in saucepan, heat, add salt and serve.

Turkey-Potato Soup

2 cups turkey or chicken broth
  prepared as above recipe
1 cup turkey or chicken meat
1 Irish potato, with skin

1 small onion, diced
1 small can mushrooms
Dash salt

Place first 5 ingredients in blender, blending well. Place in saucepan, add salt, heat, and serve.

Fish Broth

Keep the fish head, tail, fins, skin and bones for stock. Partly cover with cold water. Add cut-up vegetables suitable for soup:

1 onion   Celery stalk with leaves
1/2 carrot   Seasonings to taste

Simmer the stock for about 1/2 hr. Strain. Serve as soup, or use it in aspic or sauces. The stock may be kept for several days in tightly closed container in the refrigerator.

Roman Egg Soup

1 qt. chicken broth   1/8 tsp. salt
4 eggs, beaten until thick   1/8 tsp. pepper
1-1/2 tbsp. whole wheat flour
1-1/2 tbsp. parmesan cheese,
   grated

Bring chicken broth to boiling point, add egg slowly, until well blended. Continue stirring and add remaining ingredients. Let simmer for about 5 min.

Hot Mushroom Soup

2 cups meat or vegetable stock   2 med. potatoes, scrubbed and
2 cups mushrooms   cubed
1 small onion   1 tsp. marjoram

Put all ingredients in blender or food grinder; whip or chop fine. But 1 tbsp. cooking oil in a heavy saucepan, add the soup mixture, season with sea kelp and simmer about 5 min. Put in thermos bottle for the lunch, if need be.

Creamed Alfalfa Sprout Soup

1 qt. water
3/4 cup raw cashew nuts
2 tbsp. arrowroot powder
1 tbsp. whole wheat pastry
  flour

2 tsp. salt
1 tsp. onion powder
1/2 tsp. celery seed powder
2 tbsp. Energy broth
1 cup alfalfa sprouts

Liquefy first 8 ingredients, then bring to a boil and cook until it thickens. Chop alfalfa sprouts, approx. 1/4 cup to each bowl, and add just before serving. Serves 3-4.

Parlsey Vegetable Broth

1 bunch parsley
1 small onion
1 tbsp. butter
1/4 cup vegetable broth
  powder

1 bunch spinach
1 small carrot
2 cups celery, chopped
Parsley sprigs

Wash spinach and celery, chop very fine. Grate onion and carrot. Combine and cover with water. Cook slowly for 20 min. Season with butter and broth powder, sprinkle with chopped parsley and serve.

Tomato Soy Bean Broth

1 cup cooked soy beans
1 small onion, cut fine

4 cups tomato juice
2 small green peppers, cut fine

Steam onion and green pepper 10 min. Add mashed soy beans and tomato juice. Heat, but do not boil. Dot with butter and serve.

Tomato-Almond-Asparagus Soup

4 to 6 cooked asparagus spears
1 No. 2 can tomatoes
1 cup raw almonds
1 vine-ripened tomato, if
   desired

Dash onion salt
Dash vegetable salt

Place first 4 ingredients in blender, blending well. Add salts and heat, but do not boil.

Tomato-Cashew Soup

1 No. 2 can tomatoes
1/2 bunch parsley
1 tsp. minced onion

1/2 cup raw cashews
Dash vegetable salt

Place first 4 ingredients in blender and blend well. Add salt and heat, serving immediately.

Swedish Cucumber Soup

4 cups buttermilk
1 cup sour cream
1 cup cucumber, diced
1/2 cup cooked beet greens,
   finely chopped

1 tbsp. raw carrot, grated
1 tbsp. onion, finely chopped
1 tbsp. dill
1/4 tsp. pepper
1 tsp. salt

Beat buttermilk and sour cream until smooth, add vegetables and seasonings. Simmer gently until vegetables are tender. Do not boil. Serves 6-8. In summer chill this soup without simmering, and serve very cold.

Frozen Pea-Tomato Soup

4 med. vine-ripened tomatoes	Dash of salt
2 stalks celery, large	1 pkg. frozen peas
1/2 cup almonds, raw	1/2 tsp. butter
1/2 tsp. onion, grated	1/2 cup water

Defrost peas until they separate. Place all ingredients, except butter and salt, in blender, blending well. Add salt and butter and heat. Do not boil. Serve immediately.

CHAPTER 10: MENUS

Special breakfast, luncheon and dinner suggestions have been given separately in the readings. Following these, readings giving a whole day's menus will be given. At the conclusion of this section, we will give a few menus prepared for the average daily diet by nutritional authorities.

Before considering the readings' breakfast suggestions, remember that in recent years nutritionists have become very much concerned with the bad breakfast patterns in this country. They point out that breakfast is extremely important, and that a toast-coffee-and-orange juice breakfast can have a bad effect upon the body's capacity for morning energy. Researchers at Marquette University say that temperatures inside the stomach drop when one is hungry, but are quickly restored to normal after eating. At 11 o'clock, they say, the poor breakfasters first feel hungry. The temperature drops, and this leads to a lowering of metabolism in the stomach. Doctors believe that this means lower body fires. Accordingly, 11A.M. is the hour of lowered vitality for many, many people.

In the mornings, eat a whole-grain cereal, well cooked, with milk or cream; or eat citrus fruits. Do not take the citrus fruits and the cereals at the same meal. Rather, alternate these from day to day. Rice cakes, corn cakes or the like, with syrup or honey are well to be taken occasionally. 2693-P-1

In the mornings, eat citrus fruits, preferably with the pulp—having oranges at times, lemons at times, and grapefruit at other times. Then have whole wheat toast or cakes with milk, and use honey as the sweetening. At other times, eat cooked whole wheat cereal or Wheaties, Grape Nuts or any of those that carry a great deal of

153

iron and vitamins for the system. But do not give cereals and fruit juices or citrus fruit, at the same meal.

318-P-5

In the mornings, eat citrus fruit or stewed fruits such as figs, apples, peaches or the like. But do not serve the stewed fruits with the citrus fruit juices, nor the citrus fruits with a dry cereal . . . when cereals are taken, there may be added buckwheat cakes, rice cakes, or a coddled egg, and a cereal drink. It would be well for these to be altered or changed occasionally. 623-P-1

Don't be satisfied with just taking a sandwich for lunch. Use only green vegetables or fresh green vegetables in the lunch period. Don't just eat a scrap of bread and a scrap of meat, or a chocolate soda, or a milk shake. These are poisons for the system at such periods. 243-P-11

At noon, eat a green vegetable diet, without too much bread. Eat brown bread at such times. These vegetables may be seasoned with oils or dressings. Eat vegetable soups, mostly made with green vegetables. Or eat meat soups, but none of the heavier foods. 943-P-8

For lunch, eat rather lightly. For sweets, take the fruit juices or pies with milk. 781-P-1

At noon, eat some raw vegetables such as lettuce, celery, carrots or the like; with some soup, preferably vegetable soup. 2693-P-1

At noon, eat green vegetables, such as carrots, cabbage, slaw, lettuce, celery, spinach and the like. These should be taken preferably with oil dressings. At this meal, there may also be taken at times . . . meat juices but no meats. 623-P-1

In the evenings, eat meat in moderation, but no red meat, and no hog meats at any time, although very crisp bacon may be eaten at times with eggs. But do not have any grease in it. . . . Drink plenty of water during the whole day. 943-P-8

154

In the evenings, do not eat too heavily. Eat fish, fowl or lamb—although they should never be fried. Have well-cooked vegetables. This is not all that may be eaten, but it is an outline.   2693-P-1

In the evening, eat meat but not too much; and a well-balanced vegetable diet of those that grow above the ground.   781-P-1

This would be given as an outline [of the day's foods]; not as the only foods, but as an outline:

Mornings: Whole grain cereals or citrus fruit juices though not at the same meal. When using orange juice, combine lime with it. When using grapefruit juice, combine lemon with it. Have an egg, preferably only the yolk; or rice or buckwheat cakes; or toast. Any one of these would be well in the mornings.

Noons: A raw salad, including tomatoes, radishes, carrots, celery, lettuce, watercress—any or all of these; with a soup or vegetable broth; or sea foods.

Evenings: Fruits, such as cooked apples; potatoes, tomatoes; fish, fowl or lamb—and occasionally beef but not too often. Keep these as the main part of a well-balanced diet.   1523-P-9

In the matter of diet, we would have this as an outline; though, to be sure, this may be alternated from time to time to suit the tastes of the body. At least 3 mornings each week, we would have rolled or cracked whole wheat that is not cooked too long so that the whole vitamin force is destroyed. This will add to the body the proper portions of iron, silicon and the vitamins necessary to build up the blood supply that makes for resistance in the system.

We at other times would have citrus fruits, citrus fruit juices, the yolk of eggs, preferably soft-boiled or coddled—not the white portions; browned bread with butter;

Ovaltine or milk or coffee (provided there is no milk or cream in same). Occasionally have stewed figs, stewed raisins, prunes or apricots. But do not eat citrus fruits at the same meal with cereals, or gruels, or any of the breakfast foods.

Noons: Preferably eat raw fresh vegetables, none cooked at this meal . . . tomatoes, lettuce, celery, spinach, carrots, beet tops, mustard, onions, or the like that make for purifying in the lymph blood. We would not take any quantity of soups or broths at noon.

Evenings: Broths or soups may be taken in a small measure; but let it consist principally of vegetables that are well cooked; and a little of meats such as lamb, fish, fowl. These are preferable. No fried foods.   840-P-1

This is not all that is to be taken, but is given as an outline:

Mornings: Citrus fruit juices. When orange juice is taken, add lime or lemon juice to it, four parts orange juice to one part lime or lemon. When other citrus fruits are taken, such as pineapple or grapefruit, they may be taken as they are from the fresh fruit . . . a little salt added, if preferable. Take whole wheat bread, toasted, with butter. Coddled egg, only the yolk of same. A small piece of very crisp bacon, if so desired. Any or all of these may be taken. But when cereals are taken, do not have citrus fruits at the same meal! Such a combination produces just what we are trying to prevent in the system. When cereals are used, have either cracked wheat or whole wheat, or a combination of barley and wheat as in Maltex, if these are desired. Or Puffed Wheat, Puffed Rice, or Puffed Corn—any of these. And these may be taken with certain kinds of fresh fruits, such as berries of any nature—even strawberries if desired—no, they won't cause any rash if they are taken properly! Or peaches. The sugar used should be saccharin or honey. A cereal drink may be had if desired.

Noons: Only raw, fresh vegetables. All of these may be

combined, but grate them and don't eat them so hurriedly that they would make for that unbalanced condition (resulting from) improper mastication. Each time you take a mouthful, it should be chewed at least 4 to 20 times . . . each should be chewed so that there is the opportunity for the flow of the gastric forces from the salivary glands to be well mixed with same. Then we will find that these foods will make for bettered conditions in the body.

Evenings: Vegetables that are cooked in their own juices; each cooked alone, then combined afterward if so desired by the body. These may include any of the leafy vegetables or any of the bulbar vegetables; but cook them in their own juices! There may be meats, if so desired, or there may be added—if preferred—the proteins that come from the combination of other vegetables . . . in the forms of a certain character of pulse, or of grains.   No. 3823-P-2

Mornings: Citrus fruits, either cereals or fruits . . . or have citrus fruits and a little later have rice cakes or buckwheat or graham cakes, with honey in the honeycomb; and with milk—preferably the raw milk if it is certified milk!

Noons: Rather vegetable juices than meat juices; with raw vegetables—a salad or the like.

Evenings: Vegetables, with such as carrots, peas, salsify, red cabbage, yams or white potatoes. These potatoes should be the smaller variety and if eaten with the jackets it will be better. Then the finishing, or dessert . . . blanc mange, or jello, or jellies with fruits such as peaches, apricots, fresh pineapple or the like.
These foods, as we find, with the occasional eating of sufficient meat for strength, would bring a well-balanced diet. Occasionally we would add those foods of a blood-building type, once or twice a week: the pig knuckles, tripe, calves' liver, or such meats as brains and the like.   275-P-21

Question: Outline diet for 3 meals a day that would be best for this body.

Answer: Mornings: Citrus fruit juices or cereals, but not both at the same meal. [Use with] other cereals at times, dried fruits or figs combined with dates and raisins— these chopped very well together. And, for this special body, a mixture of dates and figs that are dried, cooked with a little corn meal (a very little sprinkled in—) then this taken with milk . . . should be almost a spiritual food for this body. Whether it's taken one, two, three or four meals a day. This is to be left to the body itself to decide.

Noons: Foods such as vegetable juices . . . and a combination of raw vegetables. But not ever any acetic acid or vinegar or the like with same. Oils, if they are olive oil or vegetable oils, may be used with same.

Evenings: Vegetables that are of the leafy nature; fish, fowl or lamb preferably, as meats—or their combinations. These of course are not to be all the foods, but this is the general outline for the three meals for the body.

275-P-34

Mornings: Whole wheat toast, brown bread; cereals with fresh fruits. The citrus fruit juices occasionally. But do not mix the citrus fruit juices and cereals at the same meal.

Noons: Principally (very seldom deviating from these) raw vegetables or raw fruits made into a salad. Not having the fruits and vegetable combined, but these may be varied. Use such vegetables as cabbage cut very fine; carrots, spinach, celery, onions, tomatoes, radishes; any or all of these. It is preferable that they all be grated, but when they are grated, do not discard the juices. These should be used upon the salad itself (from the fruits, on the fruit salad; from the vegetables on the vegetable salad). . . .

Preferably use oil dressings, such as olive oil with paprika. Even egg—that is, the yolk—may be included in these same dressings. Work the yolk of a hard-boiled egg into the oil as a portion of the dressing. . . . Use in fruit salad such fruits as bananas, papaya, guava, grapes, all kinds of fruits except apples. Apples should only be eaten when cooked, preferably baked and served with butter or hard sauce on same, topped with cinnamon and spice.

Evenings: A well-balanced cooked vegetable diet, including principally those things that will make for iron to be assimilated in the system.   935-P-1

For the purposes of comparison, let us consider a day's menu suggested in the booklet, *Recommended Dietary Allowances,* National Research Council, Number 129, page 26. This menu fulfills recommended dietary allowances for a "physically active man."

BREAKFAST

Menu 1	*Menu 2*
Orange Juice	Tomato juice
Cooked cereal, milk	Ready-to-eat cereal, milk
Eggs	Eggs
Toast, butter or margarine	Hot biscuits, butter or
Beverage	fortified margarine
	Jelly
	Beverage

LUNCH

Baked macaroni and tomatoes	Baked sweet potato
Green beans	Turnip greens or collards
Rolls, butter or fortified margarine	Sliced onions with vinegar
Fruit in season	Corn bread or muffins, butter or fortified margarine
Milk	Molasses
	Beverage

DINNER

Menu 1	*Menu 2*
Broiled chopped steak	Fried fish
Creamed potatoes, carrots	Hominy grits, cole slaw
Head lettuce,	Bread, butter or
French dressing	fortified margarine
Bread, butter or	Stewed prunes or fruit in
fortified margarine	season
Apple pie and cheese	Cookies—beverage
Beverage	

Some Menus Suggested for Chidren

Question: I would appreciate an outline of an ideal daily diet for this child's age (6 years) and for the near future.

Answer: Mornings—Whole grain cereals or citrus fruits, but these never taken at the same meal. Rather, alternate these, using one on one day and the other the next, and so on. Any form of rice cakes or the like; the yolk of eggs and the like.

Noons—Some fresh raw vegetable salad, including many types. Soups with brown bread, or broths or such.

Evenings—A fairly well-coordinated vegetable diet, with three vegetables above the ground to one below the ground. Sea food, fowl or lamb; not other types of meats. Gelatine may be prepared with any of the vegetables—as in the salads for the noon meal—or with milk and cream dishes. These would be well for the body. 3224-P-2

For a nine-year-old:

160

In the evenings, eat a great deal of whole vegetables, well balanced with meats. Eat all the leafy vegetables that agree with the body. And let several of the evening meals each week contain calf's liver, hog tripe, beef tripe, or the like. Do not give the body hog meats. . . . Drink as much milk as the body may well take at such meals. . . . At noon, eat a great deal of butter and bread, or those foods that carry a high calorie content in carbohydrates, or sweets, provided they are honey-based. For honey will act with the digestive forces in the system much better than corn or cane sweets.   318-P-5

For a six-month-old baby:

Do not overcrowd the stomach or be over-anxious as to the amount [of food] taken, especially through the hot months. . . . Have plenty of fruit juices—that is, orange juice, preferably, then other juices as the body develops. But do not overcrowd these through the hot months. Make the changes more in the early fall, but not . . . too much in the present.

Also have plenty of strained oatmeal, but not on the same days when the orange juice is given. Use preferably the steel-cut oats, strained, and with plenty of milk.

Yes, owing to the general strength and tendency of the body in the bone structure, there is the inclination for not sufficient calcium. Thus it would be well for the body to have the Haliver Oil rather than the cod liver oil. This . . . in the form of pellets. . . . The body will be able to take it without choking, provided it is given at meals.
                                                    2289-P-1

For all growing bodies:

In general conditions, you must know that there is a growing body and that there is necessarily . . . (much) activity and that the energies must be supplied. Also, there is a drain upon the whole of the nerve and blood supply of the body. Hence, meat should be a portion of the diet each day, though it should not be the greater portion, and it need not be eaten at every meal.

759-P-7

CHAPTER 11: QUESTIONS ABOUT SPECIFIC FOODS AND COOKERY—FOOD ELEMENTS

Steam pressure and waterless cooking are the modern methods advised nowadays for preservation of maximum vitamin and mineral content. The use of Patapar paper accomplishes the same end. This is not now manufactured, we understand, but a similar paper may be obtained from the Kalamazoo Vegetable Parchment Co., Kalamazoo, Michigan.

Keep away from heavy foods. Use those which are body-building, such as beef broth, beef juices, liver, fish and lamb. Never eat fried foods. Include butter and milk and raw vegetables; preparing the latter often with gelatin. Eat only the yolk of the egg. Leafy vegetables are all right—raw cabbage and cooked red cabbage, spinach and string beans. But not dry beans, nor white potatoes, and only a few sweet potatoes and yams. Artichokes are all right in season, but prepare them in Patapar paper, so that the juices mix with the pulp.   7059-P-1

Question: How about steam pressure for cooking foods quickly? Does it destroy any of the vitamins of the vegetables and fruits?

Answer: No, it preserves rather than destroys them.
                                                      462-P-5

Question: Does Steam Pressure cooking at 15 pounds temperature destroy food values in vegetables?

Answer: No. [Retention of food values] depends upon preparation, the age and how long since gathered. All these are factors affecting food values. Just as it is so well advertised that coffee loses its value in fifteen to twenty or twenty-five days after being roasted; so do foods or vegetables lose their food values after being gathered—in the same proportion in hours, as coffee does in days. 340-P-30

In the matter of the diet throughout the periods of convalescence, we would constantly add more and more of Vitamin B-1, in every form in which it may be taken: in bread, in cereals, in types of vegetables . . . in fruits, etc. Be sure that there is sufficient each day of B-1 for adding to the vital energies. These vitamins are not stored in the body as A, D, and O, but it is necessary to add these daily. All of those fruits and vegetables that are yellow in color should be taken: oranges, lemons, grapefruit, yellow squash, yellow corn, yellow peaches—also beets. *But all of the vegetables should be cooked in their own juices, and the body should eat the juices with same.* 2529-P-1

On the subject of tomatoes, which many people say are too "acid" for their particular systems, the readings shed considerable light.

Question: What is the effect on my system of eating so many tomatoes?

Answer: Quite a dissertation might be given as to the effect of tomatoes upon the human system.

Of all the vegetables, tomatoes carry most of the vitamins, in a well-balanced assimilable manner suitable for the activities in the system. Yet if these tomatoes are not cared for properly, they may become very destructive to a physical organism. That is, if they ripen after being pulled, or if there is contamination with other influences or substances.

In this particular body, as we find, the reactions from tomatoes have not always been the best. Neither has there been a normal reaction from eating same. For here there is a tendency to make for irritation or humour. Nominally, though, tomatoes should form at least a portion of a meal three or four days out of every week, and they will be found most helpful. . . . The tomato is one vegetable that in most instances . . . is preferable to be eaten after being canned, for it is then much more uniform. The reaction from non-canned tomatoes in this body, then, has been to form an acid of its own; though the tomato is among those foods which may be termed non-acid forming. 584-P-5 (10/4/1935)

Question: Would it be well for me to eat vegetables such as corn, tomatoes, and the like?

Answer: Corn and tomatoes are excellent. More of the vitamins are obtained from tomatoes than from any other growing vegetable. 180-P (5/26/1928)

It will be very interesting and instructive to compare the food values attributed by the readings to certain foods with a similar listing given by any textbook on nutrition or leaflets obtainable from the National Research Council; Metropolitan Life Insurance Company; National Livestock and Meat Board; and the U. S. Department of Agriculture. Verification will be found for the information given in the Edgar Cayce readings—in many instances, many years before food facts were established by modern research.

Question: Should plenty of lettuce be eaten?

Answer: Plenty of lettuce should always be eaten by almost everybody, for this supplies an effluvium in the blood stream that is a destructive force for most of those influences that attack the blood stream. It's a purifier.
404-P-4

Keep plenty of those foods that supply calcium to the body. These we would find especially in raw carrots, cooked turnips and turnip greens, and all kinds of salads—especially of watercress, mustard greens and the like; these especially taken raw, though turnip greens cooked, but cooked in their own juices and not with fat meats. 1968-P-2

Often use the raw vegetables which are prepared with gelatin. Use them at least three times each week. Those which grow more above the ground than those which grow below the ground. Do include, when they are prepared, the carrots with that portion especially close to the top. It may appear the harder and less desirable, but it carries the vital energies (which) stimulate the optic reactions between kidneys and the optics.   3051-P

Keep away from sweets, especially chocolates at this period; also foods prepared with coconut. Other kinds of nuts are well, and almonds are especially good. An almond a day is much more in accord with keeping the doctor away, especially certain types of doctors, than apples! ... For the apple was the fall ... remember, the almond blossomed when everything else died.   3180-P-2

In connection with almonds, which have food values little considered even by those in the field of nutrition, it is quite interesting to note how the readings' information tallies with the latest research and investigation. In *Recommended Dietary Allowances* by the National Research Council, page 17, it is stated that "In the case of other adults the phosphorus allowances should be approximately 1.5 times those for calcium." According to the USDA Handbook No. 8, *Composition of Foods, Raw, Processed and Prepared*, almonds are at the top of the list of foods having such a proportion of phosphorus and calcium. Almonds contain 475 Mg. of Phosphorus, 254 Mg. of Calcium—and in addition 4.4 Mg. of iron. *Almonds rank highest in iron of all foods having the proportion of 1.5 phosphorus to amount of calcium.*

Question: Please give foods that supply iron, calcium and phosphorus.

Answer: Cereals that carry the heart of the grain; vegetables of the leafy kinds, fruits and nuts. *The almond carries more phosphorus and iron in a combination easily assimilated, than any other nut.*   1131-P-2

For supplying the system with calcium and other elements, such as phosphorus and salts ... eat sea foods at least once or twice a week, especially clams, oysters, shrimp or lobster. The oyster or clam often taken raw; the others roasted or boiled, seasoned with butter.

275-P-21

The phosphorus-forming foods are principally carrots, lettuce (rather the leaf lettuce, which has more soporific activity than the head lettuce), shell fish, salsify, the peelings of white potatoes (if they are not too large potatoes).

560-P-1

Vitamins—should we take them separately or in foods? The Edgar Cayce readings varied in their advice, apparently according to the individual's body capacities. In the majority of readings, however, the position was taken that it is better to obtain the vitamins from foods.

So keep an excess of foods that carry vitamins, especially Vitamin B, iron and such. Do not take the concentrated form of vitamins, you see, but obtain these from foods. These foods would include all fruits, all vegetables that are yellow ... thus lemon and orange juice combined; all citrus fruit juices, pineapple as well as grapefruit. Some of these should be a part of the diet each day. Squash, especially the yellow; carrots, cooked and raw; yellow peaches; yellow apples—preferably have the apples cooked. All of these carry an excess of the greater quantity of the necessary elements for supply of energies for the body and are more easily assimilated by the body. Yellow corn, yellow corn meal, buckwheat—all are especially good; also red cabbage. Such vegetables, such fruits, are especially needed for the body of this individual.

1968-P-3

Knowing the tendencies (toward weakness in your body), supply in the vital energies that which ye call vitamins or elements. For remember, though we may give many combinations (for treatments), there are only four elements in your body: water, salt, soda and iodine. These are the basic elements; they make all the rest! Each vitamin, as a component part of an element, is simply a

167

combination of these other influences—given a name, mostly for confusion, by those who would tell you what to do, for a price!   2533-L-4

All such properties as vitamins that add to the system are more efficacious if they are given for periods, left off for periods, and then begun again. For if the system comes to rely upon such influences wholly, it ceases to produce the vitamins, even though the food values are kept normally balanced. It is much better for these vitamins to be produced in the body from the normal development than supplied mechanically, for nature is much better, still, than science! As we find, then, these vitamins should be given twice a day for two to three weeks; left off for a week, and then begun again, especially through the winter months. This method would be much more effective with the body.   759-P-10

Question: What relationships do vitamins bear to the glands? Give specific vitamins affecting specific glands.

Answer: You want a book written on this subject! They—the vitamins—are food for the glands. Vitamins are that from which glands take those influences necessary to supply energies, to enable various organs of the body to reproduce themselves. Would you ever consider it likely that the toenails would reproduce themselves by the influences of the same gland which supplies the breast—or head, or face? Or that the cuticle would be supplied from the same source which supplies the organ of the heart itself?

These [building substances] *are taken from glands* controlling assimilated foods; hence foods require elements or vitamins to supply various forces enabling each organ and function of organ, in the whole body, to carry on its creative and generating force, see?

In discussing the vitamins, let us being with A. It supplies portions of the nerves—to the bone and to the brain itself. It is not all of the supply to this area, but this is a part of the function of A vitamin.

Then vitamin B and B-1 supply energies, or the moving forces of the nerve and white blood supply, for itself, and the brain for itself. These [vitamins] supply the sympathetic or involuntary reflexes through the body. And this [energy] includes all kind—whether you are wriggling your toes, or ears, or batting your eyes, or whatever!

In these [B vitamins] we also have that influence which supplies the chyle with its ability to control the use of fats.—This body has never had enough of it; and this [control of use of fats] is necessary for carrying on the reproducing of oils which prevent tenseness in joints, or prevent joints from becoming dry or atrophied—seeming to creak. At times, the body has had some creaks!

In vitamin C we find that which supplies influences necessary for the flexes of every nature throughout the body: of a muscular or tendon nature; a heart reaction; a kidney contraction; a liver contraction or the opening or shutting of your mouth or batting of the eye, or supplying of the saliva, and the muscular forces in the face. These are all supplied by vitamin C. Not that C is the only supply, but it forms a part of it.

C is that from which the [necessary supplies for] structural portions of the body are [taken and] stored; then drawn upon when it becomes necessary. And when [lack of C] has become detrimental to the body—which has been the case for this body—it is necessary to supply vitamin C in such proportions as to aid. Else conditions become such that bad eliminations result, because of incoordination between excretory functions of the alimentary canal—as well as functioning of the heart, liver and lungs—through the expelling of forces that are a part of the structural portion of the body.

Vitamin G supplies the general energies, or the sympathetic forces of the body itself. These are some of the principles.   2072-P-5

Question: What foods carry most of the Vitamin B?

Answer: All those that are of the yellow variety, especially, and whole-grain cereals or bread.   457-P-4

In the matter of diet throughout the periods of (convalescence), we would constantly add more and more of vitamin B-1, in every form in which it may be taken: in bread, in cereals, in types of vegetables . . . fruits, etc. Be sure that each day there is sufficient vitamin B-1 to add vital energies, for B vitamins are not stored in the body, as are A, D, and G. It is necessary to add these daily. All those fruits and vegetables, then, that are yellow should be taken: oranges, lemons, grapefruit, yellow squash, yellow corn, yellow peaches . . . beets. But all of the vegetables should be cooked in their own juices, and the body should take the juices along with vegetables.

2529-P-1

What are vitamins? One scientist of note has said that a vitamin is a unit of ignorance—nobody knows what it is, only what it does. Listen to the Cayce reading:

Have ye not read that in Him ye live and move and have thy being? What are those elements in food or in drink that give growth or strength to the body? Vitamins? What are vitamins? The Creative Forces working with body-energies for the renewing of the body! 3511-P-1

And again:

Know that the body must function as a unit. One person may get his feet wet and have a cold in the head. Another may get his head wet and have a cold. The same is true in any relationship. For in the body, the circulation carries within the corpuscles such elements or vitamins as may be needed for assimilation in each organ. Each organ has within itself a special ability to create from what is assimilated the elements needed to build itself. . . Hence it may be said that the adding of vitamins to the system is merely a precautionary measure at seasons when the body is the most susceptible to colds—either by contact, by exposure, or from unsettled conditions.   7046-L-1

Remember your high school days in chemistry class, when you added a "catalyst" to the chemicals with which you were working, and their reaction was speeded up amazingly? The newly emphasized *amino acids,* with which scientific literature is filled now, seem—at least to an informed layman—to be such catalysts. The various kinds of amino acids, when isolated and tested, always seem to be needed by certain vitamins so that the action of the vitamins can be more fully realized by the body.

This new emphasis on amino acids takes on new significance in the light of the Cayce reading on diet, especially with regard to gelatin. You have noticed how often gelatin was mentioned and recommended. Over ten years ago, someone asked the sleeping Cayce:

Question: Please explain the vitamin content of gelatin. There is no reference to vitamin content on the package.

Answer: It isn't the vitamin content in gelatin (which is important), but its ability to *work with* the activities of the glands. It enables the glands to take from what has been absorbed or digested the vitamins—otherwise inactive if it were not for sufficient gelatin in the body. There may be mixed with any chemical, you see, that which would make the system able to use what is present and needed. The system becomes, then, as it were, "sensitive" to conditions. Without it [the gelatin] there is not that sensitivity [to vitamins].   849-P-6

We quote from the *Gelatin Guide—What Gelatin Is and How to Use It,* obtained from the Knox Gelatine Company:

"No one food article supplies all of the types of amino acids that make up the complete protein. . . . Real gelatin and several of the cereal and vegetable proteins are in this class. Unflavored gelatin which contains 9 of the 10 essential amino acids takes its place as a useful supplementary protein. . . . The protein of real gelatin contains amino acids that have special value in the production of hemoglobin." . . . Protein must also serve as

171

material for the precursors of essential biological catalysts such as enzymes and hormones."

Food and Nutrition News, published by the National Live Stock and Meat Board, stated as far back as October 1952: "Research indicates that the requirement or metabolism of all vitamins is interrelated with that for protein or specific amino acids. One nutrient can no longer be considered apart from all other nutrients."

Not too heavy a diet; that is, not too much meats, more vegetables. Fruits and nuts may be included . . . raw vegetables prepared oft with gelatin. Gelatin, ices, ice cream: all of these may be taken.   3395-P-1

Do not leave off the gelatin. Do keep the vitamins that will add strength to the body.   3389-P-1

Do have raw vegetables oft. These not as to cause too great a relaxation, but [to obtain] those energies as with the nerve-building forces from celery, lettuce, tomatoes, carrots . . . but grated or chopped fine. Oft prepare these with gelatin.   5246

In the diet of this body, keep plenty of raw vegetables such as watercress, celery, lettuce, tomatoes and carrots. Change the manner of preparation of these, but do have some of these each day. They may be prepared rather often with gelatin, such as lime or lemon gelatin, or Jello. These will not only taste good but be good for you.
          3429-P-1

Have a great deal of such foods as liver, tripe, pig's knuckle, pig's feet and the like; a great deal of okra and its products; a great deal of any kind of desserts carrying quantities of gelatin. Any of the gelatin products, though they may carry sugars at times, should be had often in the diet.   2520-P-1

In building up the body with foods, preferably have a great deal of raw vegetables for this body: as lettuce, celery, carrots, watercress. All should be taken raw, with

172

dressing, and often with gelatin. The vegetables should be grated or cut very fine—even ground; but do preserve all of the juice with them, when they are prepared in this manner with gelatin.   5394-P-1

CHAPTER 12: MISCELLANEOUS HEALTH INFORMATION

So far as we know, the science of modern dietetics has done no research on the subject of acclimatization by means of using foods grown in the specific locality to which the individual wishes to become quickly adjusted. Acclimatization itself has not been defined, nor have any difficulties or diseases been traced to the lack of it. Those who travel to other sections of the country—or even a few miles beyond home territory—are commonly heard to complain of the upset caused by a change of drinking water. Such an upset may just as easily be caused by change of food grown in another locality, reacting differently in the body.

The Edgar Cayce readings have very definite advice to give on the subject of acclimatization. The reader may find a fertile and fascinating subject for speculation in the fact that frozen foods, vegetables, meats and sea foods native to specific sections are widely used in many other sections of the country. Is there any connection between this fact and the enormous trek to Florida, California and adjacent parts of the country? Is the consumption of such foods helping to make us more national minded? Is it sweeping away some of the sectional prejudices? Is it making us more nomadic?

Question: Is the climate of Austin, Texas, satisfactory and should I remain here?

Answer: The climatic conditions here are not the basis of the trouble. The body can adjust itself. As we have indicated, bodies can usually adjust themselves to climatic conditions if they adhere to the proper diet and activities, or eat all characters of foods that are produced in the area where they reside. This will more quickly adjust a body to any particular area or climate than any other thing.

Question: Is a diet composed mainly of fruits, vegetables, eggs and milk the best diet for me?

Answer: As indicated, use more of the products of the soil that are grown in the immediate vicinity. These are better for the body than any specific set of fruits, vegetables, grasses, or what not. We would add more of the original sources of proteins.   4047-P-1

Have vegetables that are fresh and especially those grown in the vicinity where the body resides. Shipped vegetables are never very good.   2-P-14

Have raw vegetables also, but not a great quantity of melons of any kind, though cantaloupes may be taken if grown in the neighborhood where the body resides. If a cantaloupe is shipped, don't eat it. Fruits that may be taken are plums, pears, and apples—not raw apples but plenty of roasted apples.   5097-P-1

Do not have large quantities of any fruits, vegetables or meats that are not grown in or come from the area where the body is at the time it partakes of such foods. This will be found to be a good rule to be followed by all. This prepares the system to acclimate itself to any given territory.   3542-P-1

Body's Need for Water

Do you drink enough water? Most people do not drink as much as they think—or say—they do. Some health information sources say to drink six to eight glasses of water a day, exclusive of juices, tea, coffee, etc.; others lower this to four to six glasses. The practice of giving babies water in addition to milk is frowned upon nowadays—milk is mostly water, pediatricians explain. Is drinking water important and why? The Edgar Cayce readings say it is.

There should be more water taken into the system in a

more consistent manner, so that the system—especially in the hepatics and kidneys—may function normally, thus producing . . . correct elimination of drosses in the system, and for this reason each channel should be kept in equilibrium (with the other channels) so that there is not an . . . accentuated condition in any one of the eliminating functions. There should not be an overtaxing of the lungs, kidneys, liver nor respiratory, but all should be kept in an equal manner. . . . Lack of this water in the system creates an excess of such eliminations which normally should be cleansed through the alimentary canal and the kidneys; so that drosses are forced back into the capillary circulation.   257-P-7

Always drink plenty of water, before meals and after meals. For, as has often been given, when any food value enters the stomach, it immediately becomes a storehouse or a medicine chest that may create all the elements necessary for proper digestion within the system. If foods are first acted upon by pure water, the reactions are more nearly normal. Also, therefore, each morning upon arising, first take a half to three-quarters of a glass of hot water. . . Not so hot that it is objectionable. Not so tepid that it makes for sickening [reactions], but this will clarify the system of poisons.   311-MS-3

Question: How much water should I drink daily?

Answer: From six to eight tumblers full.   574-P-1

Sleep

Few of us get enough sleep; or, as much as we think or suspect we need, in order to feel at our best. If we deliberately deprive themselves of enough sleep, this will be added to our sins of neglect, or omission. The readings say, "Take Time to Sleep!"

Take time to sleep! It is the exercising of a faculty—it is a condition meant to be a part of the experience of each soul. . . . It is but the shadow of life, or lives, or experiences. Just as each day of experience is a part of the whole life that is being builded by an entity . . . [so]

176

each night is but a period of putting away—a storing up into the superconscious or the unconsciousness of the soul itself.   2067-P-1

Seven and a half to eight hours' sleep should be taken for most bodies.   816-P-1

Sedatives and hypnotics are destructive forces to brain and nerve reflexes.   3431-P-1

Question: Why can't I sleep at night?

Answer: This is from nervousness and over-anxiety. Of course, keep away from any drugs if possible—though a sedative at times may be necessary. Drink a glass of warm milk with a teaspoonful of honey stirred into it.
                                                          2514-P

Question: What may be done to enable me to sleep through the night?

Answer: Purifying of the system in the manner indicated will relieve the tension upon the nervous system. . . . For, if the body takes time for thought: physical rest is the natural means whereby the mental and spiritual forces find the means of coordination with mental-physical activities of the body. Hence rest is necessary; but that which is *induced*—unless it becomes necessary because of pain—is not a *natural rest,* nor does it produce regeneration of activities of the physical body.

                                                          1711-P-1

Question: Why am I so dependent upon sleep, and what do I do during my physical sleep?

Answer: Sleep is a *sense,* as we have given heretofore. It is that which is needed for the physical body to recuperate—or to draw from the mental and spiritual powers or forces what has been held as ideals for the body. . . . Don't think that the body is a haphazard machine, or that the things which happen to individuals are chance!

Then, what happens to a body in sleep? This depends

upon what it has thought and what it has set as its ideal. For when one considers, one may find these to be facts: there are some individuals who in their sleep gain strength, power and might, because of their thoughts, their manner of living. There are others who find that when any harm, any illness, any dejection comes to them, it is following sleep! Again, it is a law. What happens to this body? That is dependent upon the manner in which it has *applied* itself during the periods of its waking state.   2067-P

Smoking, Coffee and Tea

Is smoking permitted, or compatible with everyday living in which a strong effort is made to apply ideals? What about alcoholic drinks? Coffee and tea? Are they harmful? Information given in the readings is extremely helpful.

Question: Have personal vices such as tobacco and whiskey any influence upon one's health or longevity?

Answer: You are suffering from the use of some of these in the present, but it is over-indulgence. In moderation, these stimulants are not too bad, but man so seldom will be moderate. Or as most would say: those who indulge will make pigs of themselves. This over-indulgence, of course, makes for conditions which are to be met. For what one sows, that must one reap. This is unchangeable law.   5233

Question: Does smoking hurt the body?

Answer: Moderate smoking is not so harmful as would be the nervous and mental reaction to total abstinence from it. Six or eight (cigarettes) a day then, in moderation.   1568-P

Question: Would smoking be detrimental to me or beneficial?

Answer: This depends very much upon self. In moderation, smoking is not harmful; but to a body that holds

178

such as being out of line with its best mental or spiritual unfoldment, do not smoke.   2981-P-1

Question: Is the moderate use of liquor, tobacco and meat a bar to spiritual growth?

Answer: For this entity, yes. For some, no.   2981-L-1

Wine taken in excess, of course, is harmful. Wine taken with brown, black, rye or whole wheat bread is body-building.   821-P-1

No beer, no strong drink, though occasionally red wine may be taken as a *food*—for this is blood building, and blood forces are carried in same, such as iron and plasms that make for proper activity in the system. But never more than two or two-and-a-half ounces of same—and this only with black or brown bread, not with sweets.
                                                1308-P-1

Questions: Are too much coffee and smoking dangerous for nerves and stomach?

Answer: Not necessarily. Depends upon how the coffee is prepared—with milk or cream it can be (bad for him). Smoking in moderation is not harmful.   3477-P-1

In *Food and Nutrition News* December 1956 issue, we find this statement about coffee: "The presence of relatively large amounts of niacin, one of the B vitamins, in coffee has been confirmed by animal tests. This is relatively unimportant to Americans since their diet usually contains adequate amounts of niacin. However, among some populations abroad, the drinking of coffee may help prevent niacin deficiency."

Question: Will coffee hurt the body?

Answer: Coffee without cream or milk is not so harmful. Preferably the G. Washington Coffee for this body, because of the manner in which it is brewed.   1568-P-2

Question: Is coffee good for the body? If so, how often taken?

Answer: Coffee taken properly is a food. For many kinds of physical conditions, as with this body, caffeine in coffee is hard on the digestion—especially when there is a tendency for a plethoric condition in the lower end of the stomach. Hence the use of coffee or chicory . . . with combinations where breads, meats or sweets are taken is helpful. But for this body it is preferable that tannin (in tea) be mostly removed. Then it can be taken two or three times a day, but without milk or cream.

404-P-5

Coffee is a stimulant to the nerve system. The dross from coffee is caffeine, which is not digestible in the system and must necessarily be eliminated. Thus when caffeine is allowed to remain in the colon, poisons are thrown off from it. If it is eliminated—as it is in this system—*coffee is a food* and is preferable to many stimulants that might be taken.

294-P-37

Question: Does it hurt me to use sugar in my coffee?

Answer: Sugar is not nearly so harmful as cream. You may use sugar in moderation.

243-P-16

Coffee taken properly is a food—taken, that is, without cream or milk.

303-P

Question: Are tea and coffee harmful?

Answer: For this body, tea is preferable to coffee, but tea in excess is hard on the digestive system; to be sure, it should never be taken with milk.

1622-P-1

Question: Are tea and coffee harmful to this body?

Answer: Tea is more harmful than coffee. Any nerve reaction is more susceptible to the kind of tea that is usually found in this country, though in some ways in which it is produced, it would be well. Coffee, taken properly, is a food—that is, without cream or milk.

303-P-1

Work, rest, recreation, exercise, eliminations, food and drink—all these are the physical factors of life having mental and spiritual effects, which must be properly balanced with time we take for the purely spiritual. The difficulties of reaching this proper balance—each for himself—are reflected in the following questions put to Edgar Cayce, and the wonderfully constructive answers.

We find that these conditions arose as a result of what might be called occupational disturbances: not enough in the sun, nor enough of hard work. [There has been] plenty of brain work, but the body is supposed to coordinate the spiritual, mental and physical. He who does not give recreation a place in his life—and the proper tone to each phase—well, he just fools himself. . . . There must be certain amounts of sleep. Didn't God make man to sleep at least a third of his life? Then consider! These are physical, mental and spiritual necessities. This is what the Master meant when He said, "Consider the lilies of the field, how they grow." Do they grow all the while, bloom all the while—or look mighty messy and dirty at times? It is well for people, individuals, as this entity, to get their hands dirty in the dirt at times, and not be the white-collared man all the time! . . . From whence was man made? Don't be afraid to get a little dirt on you once in a while. . . . And take time to play a while with others. There are children growing. Have you added anything constructive to any child's life? You'll not be in heaven if you're not leaning on the arm of someone you have helped . . .   3552-P-1

Question: Do you advise the use of colonics or Epsom Salts baths for the body?

Answer: When these are necessary, yes. For everyone, everybody, should take an internal bath occasionally, as well as external baths. People would be better off if they would!   440-3

Clear the body as you do the mind of those things that have hindered. The things that hinder physically are poor eliminations. Set up better eliminations in the body. This is why osteopathy and hydrotherapy come nearer to being the basis of all needed treatments for physical disabilities.

2524-MS-2

For hydrotherapy and massage are preventive as well as curative measures. The cleansing of the system allows the bodyforces themselves to function normally and thus to eliminate poisons, congestions, and conditions that would become acute throughout the body.   257-P-51

Question: What physical and mental exercises will be beneficial?

Answer: Of course, meditation is always well—for the mental attitude has much to do with the general physical forces. As for the physical exercise: walking is the best of any exercise—and swimming now for the next three or four [warm] months.

2823-P-1

The best exercise for this body would be to stretch in the manner of a cat, or panther. Stretching the muscles but not straining them causes the tendons and muscles to be put into positions natural for the building of a strong and graceful body.

4003-P-1

Question: Is there any special exercise I should take, other than the head and neck exercise?

Answer: Walking is the best exercise, but don't take is spasmodically. Have a regular time and do it rain or shine.

No. 1968-P-4

Question: Has lack of setting-up exercises in these last months been detrimental to the body?

Answer: Whenever something is begun and then left off, it becomes detrimental—anything, that is, which should have been kept up!

457-P-7

Fasting means what the Master gave: Laying aside our own concept of *how* and *what* should be done at any period, and letting the Spirit guide. Understand the *truth* of fasting! To be sure, overindulgence in bodily appetites brings shame to self, as overindulgence in anything. True fasting is casting out of self any thought of what we would like done, and becoming *channels* for what He, the Lord, would have done in the earth through us.

395-L-2

Take time to be holy, but take time also to play. Take time to rest, time to recuperate; for thy Master, even the pattern in the earth, took time to rest. He took time to attend a wedding, took time to be apart from others, took time to attend a funeral. He took time to attend those who were awakening from death. . . . He took time to minister to all.

5246

THE A.R.E. TODAY

The Association for Research and Enlightenment, Inc., is a non-profit, open membership organization committed to spiritual growth, holistic healing, psychical research and its spiritual dimensions; and more specifically, to making practical use of the psychic readings of the late Edgar Cayce. Through nationwide programs, publications and study groups, A.R.E. offers all those interested, practical information and approaches for individual study and application to better understand and relate to themselves, to other people and to the universe. A.R.E. membership and outreach is concentrated in the United States with growing involvement throughout the world.

The headquarters at Virginia Beach, Virginia, include a library/conference center, administrative offices and publishing facilities, and are served by a beachfront motel. The library is one of the largest metaphysical, parapsychological libraries in the country. A.R.E. operates a bookstore, which also offers mail-order service and carries approximately 1,000 titles on nearly every subject related to spiritual growth, world religions, parapsychology and transpersonal psychology. A.R.E. serves its members through nationwide lecture programs, publications, a Braille library, a camp and an extensive Study Group Program.

The A.R.E. facilities, located at 67th Street and Atlantic Avenue, are open year-round. Visitors are always welcome and may write A.R.E., P.O. Box 595, Virginia Beach, VA 23451, for more information about the Association.

187